THE JOURNEY BACK

A Survivor's Guide to Leukemia

THE JOURNEY BACK

A Survivor's Guide to Leukemia

by

Jack L. Smedley

In collaboration with Iva, Scott, Karen, and Chris

© 1996 by Jack L. Smedley
Published by Rainbow's End Company
354 Golden Grove Road, Baden, Pennsylvania 15005
Printed in the United States of America

Publisher's Cataloging in Publication
(Prepared by Quality Books Inc.)

Smedley, Jack L.
    The journey back : a survivor's guide to leukemia / Jack L.
Smedley.
        p. cm.
    LCCN: 96-68497
    ISBN: 1-880451-19-0

    1. Smedley, Jack L.--Health. 2. Leukemia--Patients--
Pennsylvania--Biography.   I. Title.

RC463.S64 1996   362.1'9699419'0092
                                            QBI96-20337

Cover Design: Susan Campbell Vincent

Photo Credit: Jonathan M. Nakles

Dedication

This book is dedicated to my family who gave me the strength I needed to overcome my disease . . . especially Iva, my wife, whose optimism was, and is, never-ending.

Acknowledgments

I would like to thank Joseph Bloom, a professional editor, who took my sometimes grammatically incorrect sentences and transformed them into literary writings that will surprise and please my high school and college English instructors.

I also would like to thank Karen Towne, our family friend who, because of her personal knowledge of the events contained in this book, was able to assist me when I was searching for the right word or phrase. I think there is a professional writer inside of her, patiently waiting to surface.

Finally, my family and I would not have been in the position to write this book without the support and commitment of so many friends and other members of our family. Our triumph over my illness was supported by a network of love and, somehow, saying "thank you" just doesn't seem adequate.

Contents

FOREWARD

Y ou, the readers, have in your hands a small and powerful book that will introduce you to Jack Smedley and his family. It is my pleasure to have known Jack for over fifteen years.

Today, as busy lives are lived in frenetic times, most of us know a small amount of information about a large number of people. In years past, when people lived in close neighborhoods, small towns, or farms, they did not usually travel far. As a result, everyone ended up knowing much more about a fewer number of people. You are about to learn a lot about a man and his family—those who hold him dear and those whom he treasures. I invite you to experience and appreciate the quality time you have with the Smedleys.

In our early friendship together as busy professionals, Jack was a thoughtful, clear-thinking and trustworthy hospital administrator. When he was assigned as the hospital's representative to the University of Pittsburgh Department of Neurosurgery—of which I am chairman—the administration knew they had provided for a different level of thoughtful attention to our problems. Jack represented the promise of something extra—something more than the usual good person in a challenging job.

I remember being asked why Jack and Iva, his wife, were

invited to our departmental Christmas party since we had never previously invited a hospital administrator. I said, "Smedley is different. He is one of us. You'll see when you meet him." And so they did. You, too, will understand as you accompany him through the Valley of the Shadow.

Although Jack appears to be calm and cool, the truth is that he has a fervent, burning imagination and a creative mind. These attributes challenge him to plan and prepare thoroughly for all contingencies.

Before his bone marrow transplant, Jack devised and then carried out a planned regimen to have himself in the best possible physical, mental, emotional and spiritual condition. Jack is physically and emotionally tough. He is a man of faith—quietly but effectively living his religious beliefs. He is a truth-teller even when it is not popular to be so. He knows that success is additive—you must accomplish a series of things in the correct order if you are to succeed. Jack lives by the motto, "success is preparation." He has a sense about people that is uncanny. This is reflected in his spirit and also in his relationships with his fellowmen.

This book is about the love of a family. The power of that love is the binding thread that holds members together as they survive and triumph over Jack's life-threatening illness as well as the multiple near-death experiences that follow his bone marrow transplant. It is also about the supernatural spirit of a man who uses spiritual inner strength to control his illness and to assist in the cure of the leukemia. His struggles reflect the strong religious belief that is pervasive in his family.

This is a wonderful book about loving and about living life.

Peter J. Jannetta, M.D.
Secretary of Health for the
Commonwealth of Pennsylvania

INTRODUCTION

The prospect of dying from a life-threatening disease changes almost every aspect of an individual's life. For me the diagnosis of chronic myeloid leukemia changed my career, my personal relationship with my family and, most of all, my outlook on life.

One benefit of hearing that you have a life-threatening disease (yes, there are some benefits) is that you stop to "smell the roses." That phrase obviously includes enjoying the beauty of nature and our environment; however, even more importantly, it should include our families, our friends, and all the other people we encounter in this journey called "life." Our lives are full of high expectations. Although we take good health for granted, very few of us truly realize its importance. We *expect* to have good health, excellent careers, secure families, and the material comforts of life.

A few months ago, while eating dinner, a female friend jokingly accused me of flirting with a waitress. Although it was not appropriate at the time for me to respond, I wanted to tell her that one of the wonderful aspects of life is taking the time to get to know the many people who cross our daily paths. We become blind to many of the interesting people and things surrounding us. It is so easy to isolate ourselves to the point that our lives only involve a circle of people who share common values and interests; we become unemotional robots who have little regard for the rest of the world.

The methods I used to overcome my disease are not magical, were not discovered in a textbook, and were not learned by watching a video. Most assuredly, they are not the only ways to work toward survival. The ideas and methods are a reflection of my spirit. It is my belief that, once we begin to tap our inner strengths, we begin the process of healing. Throughout this book, you will find a common theme of the power of touch. Whether it was the loving touch of my wife, Iva, or the touch of other people who joined me on my mental journey, the healing power of the touch of those who care should never be minimized.

When I was diagnosed with leukemia it was as if every member of my family also received the same diagnosis. While they didn't have my physical symptoms, in many respects their emotional symptoms were equal to or greater than mine. Contributing to this book has been a therapeutic process for some members of my family. Knowing about and acknowledging the things that happened to me while I was at the Fred Hutchinson Cancer Research Center, putting them into perspective, and verbalizing them through the pages of this book has closed this episode of my life. My daughter Karen said, "This book gave me the opportunity to express emotions that I would have never been able to voice." In essence I believe we all found this to be true.

Cancer patients tell things to one another that they would not share with anyone else. From my discussions with other patients, I am convinced that we all possess the means to enhance and supplement the success of the current medical treatments and procedures in the fight against life-threatening illnesses.

Although I have described the complications I encountered as a bone-marrow transplant patient, these events are not presented to alarm any prospective transplant patient. Instead, it is my desire and intention to dramatize the wonderful healing and recuperative abilities of the body. My experiences are indicative of a "worst case scenario," and yet, today, I enjoy life to the fullest. I continue to be amazed by the strength of the body to survive when the mind of the patient and the support of loved ones are working in concert with God.

CHAPTER I

You Have Leukemia

It was one of many hectic work days, but it was a day that I will remember for the rest of my life. As Vice-President of Presbyterian University Hospital (PUH) in Pittsburgh, Pennsylvania, I was often confronted with unusual situations; however, the telephone call I received on August 10, 1983 began a series of events that would change my life forever. Returning to my office after a meeting, I reviewed my telephone messages and was surprised to see the name of an individual who worked as a switchboard operator at Latrobe Area Hospital—the same place I'd worked eight years prior to my employment at PUH. I remembered Bertie as always having a smile for everyone, her attitude reflecting life as a series of happy adventures. While working at Latrobe, I had made it a practice to stop by her office on my way home every night to say good-night and also to brighten my own day by encountering someone with a smile. Although I hadn't spoken to Bertie in more than three years, I welcomed the opportunity to renew contact with her. However, at the same time, I wondered why she was calling me.

The familiar voice on the other end of line was filled with anxiety. "I'm sorry for bothering you but I just had to call and make sure you are all right." She hesitated for a moment.

"For the past three nights I dreamed that you were ill—seriously ill."

"Don't apologize for calling! It's good to hear from you but I assure you that I'm fine. Just a little tired from working too many hours. But it's already Wednesday and I'm going to relax this weekend."

"I'm relieved," she said. "But, I just had to call—the dreams seemed so real."

I thanked her but continued right on with my normal routine. Amazingly, I never reflected on the call, choosing instead to rationalize away any reason for it.

At the beginning of that summer I had been the victim of a cold that lingered through July and seemed to sap my strength. It took a real effort to paint the trim on our house and, by midsummer, I still hadn't gained back my normal energy. When I finished sealing the driveway at the beginning of August, I collapsed to my knees from fatigue and weakness.

As individuals, we often think of ourselves as indestructible so, once again, I convinced myself that my continued lack of energy was a result of overwork. Then I began shutting my office door at lunch time and taking a short nap just to get through the day. Even after all these years, I don't understand why something within me refused to acknowledge that I had a problem.

On Sunday, August 14, with my fatigue increasing and the onset of pain in my chest, I continued the rationalization process. This time, however, I believed that I had probably pulled a muscle while sealing the driveway. I thought, *If I swim laps in our backyard pool, I'll loosen the pulled muscle.*

When I completed one lap of the pool, I could barely breathe and quickly went into the house and told my wife. She immediately drove me to Latrobe Area Hospital. After going through a series of tests, I noticed a buzzing among those at the nursing station. Finally, Barbara, one of the nurses I had known for many years came back to my bed and spoke with me. She appeared worried. "You have a high white blood cell count," she said.

Apprehensively, I asked, "How high?"

"Critically high!"

Critically high, my mind echoed. *What did it mean? How sick was I?*

After being admitted to the hospital for further tests, preliminary results indicated I had pneumonia in my left lung and pericarditis (inflammation around the sac of my heart). This diagnosis came about only four days after I had received the mysterious call concerning my well-being. To this day, I cannot explain my friend's knowledge of my impending health problems.

Although my condition began to improve over the next week, my white count remained high. I was discharged from the hospital with instructions to return in four days to repeat the blood studies.

One of my duties at Presbyterian University Hospital was to serve as administrative representative to the medical staff's "Cancer Committee." I therefore had some knowledge of what diagnosis was indicated by a high white blood cell count in the absence of an infection. Although I was thinking leukemia, I was continually assured by my physicians that my blood did not show immature cell types, a key indicator of this disease. The night before I was to have my next battery of blood tests, I told Iva that if the counts were still high, my physician would probably perform a bone marrow biopsy.

I returned to the hospital for the blood work and the test results indicated that my white count was still rising. My prediction was correct and I was sent immediately for a bone marrow biopsy. At this point I became a dispassionate observer to the events that were taking place in my life and within my body. I watched with little emotion or reaction as they extracted bone marrow from my sternum. The test was performed on Thursday and, since it usually takes two to three

17

days before the results are reported, Iva and I had the weekend to agonize over the possible results. On Sunday we attended our annual church picnic, but the findings of the biopsy were never far from our thoughts.

When I called on Monday for the results, the hematologist hesitated to give me the information over the phone but, after I pressed him, he said, "You have leukemia, specifically, chronic myelocytic leukemia." Hearing these words, my mind went into a state of decreased consciousness. Although I was functioning, the shock had numbed my awareness of the people and the world around me. Everything seemed distant and dreamlike. *Was this really happening to me?*

To anyone who has not experienced this type of emotional trauma, it is difficult to appreciate a state of mind that permits one to sleepwalk through life at a decreased level of alertness. My emotions and feelings were temporarily blunted to protect me from harsh reality.

Later, when the initial shock subsided, I remembered the case presentations of the Cancer Committee of people with Chronic Myelocytic Leukemia (CML); the survival time of patients was two to three years. In my case, however, because the bone marrow study indicated I had a double Philadelphia Chromosome (a specific marker identifying this type of leukemia), my predicted time of survival was only a matter of months. Most patients who are diagnosed with CML have a single Philadelphia Chromosome. A double chromosome usually indicates the impending onset of the crisis stage of the disease at which point the survival time becomes measured in weeks.

As a child I knew a neighbor boy who had been diagnosed with leukemia. During the summer, my friends and I would play ball in a field across from his house. He usually sat in a chair with a blanket over his lap watching us. I felt sorry for him and watched helplessly as he became thinner and paler with the progression of summer. When he died that fall, I thought, *He's too young to die; it's so sad.* From then on, the word leukemia, in my mind, became synonymous with death. I made an appointment with Dr. Lee Dameshek, a hematologist at PUH, to obtain a second opinion. After hearing his confirmation of my diagnosis of CML and the prognosis, Iva and I walked out of his office and into a high-rise parking garage. I remember both of us standing and looking out over the edge of garage. I thought to myself, *Our lives are also on the edge. What is going to happen to us? To me?* The two of us remained speechless for what seemed like an eternity. We were also quiet during the ride home, allowing the information to sink in and acknowledging to ourselves that our lives would never be the same.

The next day Dr. Dameshek prescribed a course of oral chemotherapy which decreased my white count to normal in a period of three weeks. Although my counts were normal, a significant number of my cells were immature cancer cells, indicating the continued presence of leukemia.

I returned to work a couple of weeks after I was discharged from the hospital. My fellow employees treated me as if I had already died. One of the realities of working in the health care field is that when you are diagnosed with cancer or some other serious illness, everyone around you seems to know your prognosis. Into my office came a stream of people shedding tears. After a particularly emotional day following my return, I went to Schenley Park—an oasis in the midst of Pittsburgh's congestion and traffic. It is one of my favorite places with its beautiful trees and long expanses of rolling lawns. I sat under a large oak tree and did my first negotiating with God, asking Him to give me ten years to raise my children. "God, if you do Your part, I'll do mine. I'll fight the disease with all my power and, if I can, I'll help other cancer victims do likewise."

The following day I went to the University of Pittsburgh Medical School Library where I read about my disease in a number of oncology text books. I wanted to know how and in what ways the disease would progress and what I could expect in the way of symptoms. When I closed the last book and walked out of the library, I began the first day of my fight against leukemia. Reading the medical books had given me the information I needed to know about my enemy.

Maybe I can't cure myself, I thought, *but I am determined to slow down the progression of this disease. The rest is up to God!*

During my career as a hospital administrator, prior to being diagnosed with leukemia, I began using relaxation techniques to deal with the stress of my position. Now I used these same techniques to create the mental state needed to visualize the struggle within my body. At first my methods were clumsy. I would relax and close my eyes and imagine the good cells in my body fighting the leukemia cells. The platelets in my blood stream were little men who looked like bandages, the red blood cells were little men carrying oxygen tanks, and the white blood cells were soldiers carrying spears. Thus began the battle within myself to keep the leukemia in check.

Three months after receiving the diagnosis, I had a second bone marrow biopsy. This time the test results showed only a single Philadelphia Chromosome. The explanation given to me was that either the original biopsy was misread or the disease had regressed to a more stable state. I believed it was the latter, and this gave me hope that I could, in my own way, gain a measure of control over my illness. For most cancer patients, the loss of control over one's life and destiny is devastating. For the moment I viewed my future with new optimism. I had now fallen into the category of patients with an expected median survival period of thirty-eight months. *But my battle was just beginning!*

CHAPTER II

A Time For Reflection

I continued in my position as Vice-President of Presbyterian University Hospital for eighteen months after first learning of my leukemia. The demands of my position, coupled with a one-hour commute to the hospital, caused me to be continually exhausted. I felt that if I changed anything in my life, I was giving in to the disease and the leukemia was winning. Because of my fatigue, I would fall asleep on the couch immediately after dinner each evening. Just getting through the day was an effort; however, somewhere and somehow, I found the reserve of energy I needed to carry me forward. Driven by the need to provide financially for my family, I could not and would not give up. For me, the acceptance phase of my illness was repeatedly interrupted by periods of denial.

During this time I lost my effectiveness in my position at the hospital. The president of the hospital later told me that in one day I had gone from being Jack L. Smedley, the Vice-President, to Jack Smedley, the patient. My physical condition, rather than the duties of my position, became the dominant topic in my business meetings. Because my peers were having difficulty dealing with my situation, the president of the hospital requested the assistance of a professional to

21

provide guidance to my fellow workers on how to relate to me. With her help, we began to work together as a management team once again.

One day, when I was exceedingly tired, the hospital hematologist, who had read my bone marrow biopsies, saw me, pulled me aside, and told me that I had no chance of beating the leukemia if I continued at my current pace. His words caused me to stop and reflect. After lunch I left the hospital and went to Phipps Conservatory, one of my favorite spots in the city. With its beautiful indoor presentations of lush tropical plants and formal gardens, the conservatory was always my destination when I needed a respite from my daily routine. Now it was a place where I began to ponder my future, contemplating the choices I needed to make in my life. While listening to the beautiful music of Handel and sitting on my favorite bench in the Orchid Room, I realized that I must make some changes.

After a great deal of thought and discussion with my wife Iva, I decided to leave my position at the hospital in early March of 1985. My plans were to begin teaching in the fall as a part-time instructor at the University of Pittsburgh Satellite Campus in our community of Greensburg. My income was drastically reduced and the financial future of our family was placed in jeopardy by this decision; however, we scaled down our expenditures and adjusted to my new income level.

This time was very difficult for me. In fact, even before I left PUH, I had started to question every aspect of my life: my relationship with God and my family, and my feelings about myself. Finally, the prospect of dying in a period of months became a reality to me and, as I began to come to grips with my illness, I decided to start to live again rather than be preoccupied with death. Looking back on this period, I realize I had made a decision to begin to rebuild my life. I set priorities and began to plan. For years, since my father's ancestry was English and my mother's was Irish, I had talked about traveling to Britain and Ireland. In the winter of 1983 I planned an eighteen-day trip for the early summer of the following year to trace our family roots. Subsequently, in May 1984, all seven of us (Iva and I, our children Scott, Karen, and Chris, and my mother and father) left for the British Isles.

Our arrival at Gatwick Airport, London was filled with excitement and anticipation. Each of us realized, to varying degrees, the importance and meaning of this trip. It may well have been the last one for us as a family. I became nauseated as soon as we arrived at the airport and, therefore, spent the first fifteen minutes of our trip vomiting in the restroom. Following this introduction to England, I lay on a bench with my family standing right beside me, waiting for me to tell them what to do next. Since I had coordinated the trip, I was "in charge." What I did was put my physical condition out of my mind so I could continue on—something that was to become a practice for me whenever I was ill.

In many ways this trip through Britain, Scotland, and Ireland seemed like a dream. For the seven of us to be together for eighteen days without conflict was in itself a miracle. It was inspirational for me to pray in some of the great churches of England, from Durham Cathedral to the tiny church in Tidswell in the Peak District. As we were flying home, my parents gave me a very emotional "thank you." I don't believe I have ever shared anything with them that they appreciated more.

A friend of mine, a psychiatrist, told me later that I have a personality that requires a continual commitment to a defined project. The planning and execution of our trip across the ocean was my first project after being told I had a potentially fatal disease. Whether these subsequent projects were improvements to the house or yard, or simply visiting friends and relatives, they were my goals. Sometimes they were things that I could do in a day; other projects would take months or years to plan and complete. Such planning caused me to look ahead rather than dwell on my disease or the uncertainty that surrounded my life. I gained mental strength through the completion of my goals. I gained control! I learned through the years that many of the limitations caused by my leukemia were self inflicted—ones that other people expected I should exhibit.

Because I enjoyed nature so much, another project that gave me a great deal of satisfaction was the construction of a pond. The project began in the summer of 1985 in a wooded section of our property where a natural spring is located. My son Chris and I constructed underground drainage pipes to divert the running spring water to a depression in the land which is surrounded by huge maple trees. During a six-year period, Chris and I, using only shovels and picks, completed the pond. As we worked together on this project, we were also building and strengthening the relationship between father and son. Prior to the transplant, much of my mental preparation was done sitting on a rock, watching the water falling into that pond and appreciating the beauty of nature. Chris said this was "Daddy's thinking place." In the solitude of this spot, I would review the pleasures of my life. Because I was satisfied with the life I had lived, my contentment and peace began to grow.

As we were flying home from a second trip to the British Isles in 1985, loaded down with souvenirs and gifts, Iva commented on the amount of merchandise we were bringing back. Laughingly, she said, "We should open a retail shop to sell British goods."

My response surprised her. "It sounds like a wonderful idea. Let's do it!"

She looked at me questioningly. "Are you serious?"

"Why shouldn't I be?"

She was cautious. "It might be too much for you!"

"Iva, I've come to terms with my physical limitations. I

realize that I can't work eight hours a day but I have to increase my activity. This could be the opportunity I've been looking for."

She gave me a supportive smile. "If . . . if . . . you're sure, then let's go for it."

I was sure. As my mental attitude stabilized and become more positive, I recognized that this had a similar affect on my body. I was becoming more optimistic about my future and what I could accomplish.

The notion of another "project" stimulated me into action as I contacted the British Trade Authority and asked them to assist me in setting up a business, importing products from the British Isles. Although I had no experience in retailing, I did have an idea of the products I wanted to merchandise in our store. As I was developing my business plan, Iva tried to encourage and support me in this new venture. Naturally, she had some doubts. It had now been two years since I had been diagnosed with leukemia. *Who could tell what the future held?*

Throughout the years, we had shared our lives with two couples who were close friends: Karen and Chris Towne, and Kathy and George Mursch. One evening, when we were all together, we began discussing the plans for the store. As my friends asked business-related questions, I answered enthusiastically, feeling very upbeat about the project. Although they listened attentively and were supportive, they seemed quieter than usual. I knew they were concerned.

Months later, as Karen and I were painting the inside of the store, I reflected back on that evening. Teasingly, I said, "All that concern made me think that the rest of you knew something that I didn't."

"What could we have known?" She waved the paint brush at me. "You and I don't have secrets!"

"Well, no one had told me when I was going to die. I thought maybe one of you had my time line."

She smiled. "No time line! We understood that you planned to go right on living. But, admit it! Even when your're in perfect health, you take on too much. Naturally, people who care about you would be concerned."

I spent the winter and spring building the shelving and racks for the sweaters, wool blankets, and other products we were going to sell. In August 1986, we opened "Smedley's British Imports." It is impossible for me to adequately describe the importance of the store in my life and in my ultimate survival. I still remember the fragrance of the wonderful mixture of English soaps and lotions, combined with the aroma of Scottish wool.

During this time I periodically began a course of oral chemotherapy whenever my white blood cells would reach a level of 40,000 (the normal range is 5,000 to 11,000). The amount of time between the cycles of chemotherapy steadily decreased as the months and years passed. Dr. Dameshek and I stopped talking about my prognosis and I just went on living.

The store was a vehicle to meet many new and interesting people, and also provided an opportunity for me to share my own good blessings in many different ways. As people in our community became aware of my illness, I would occasionally have an individual who had cancer walk into the store. Sharing his or her thoughts in regard to their spouse, children, friends, religion, and death with someone who wasn't emotionally invested in their lives, or there to make judgments, gave the person comfort and freedom. Statements could be made to me that could not have been made to family or close friends. There is a great deal to be said for "walking the same path." Sharing my optimism with these cancer patients further strengthened my own desire to hang onto life.

In particular, I recall Bob, a member of our church, who was diagnosed with cancer of the esophagus. This retired telephone worker, now tending his farm, could fix anything. If a job required two men, he would find a way to do the work

26

himself. Our pastor asked me to talk with him concerning his decision as to whether or not he would receive treatment for his cancer. When I contacted him, he said he wanted to talk to me alone.

On a very cold day in February, the two of us went outside and began walking around his lake. We discussed the options that were available to him. Though the weather didn't seem to affect Bob, I was freezing. We probably walked around the lake five or six times that day, discussing his family, death and dying, and what he would do with the cattle and farm.

"It's important to me," he said, "that I'm not helpless and pitied near the end of my life."

"I understand how you feel, "I said, looking directly into his eyes. "I've had the same concerns." And so we continued to walk and share as Bob gave verbal release to his fears and innermost thoughts. Later, I learned that whenever he was depressed—or simply needed to think about his situation— he would, in his mind, walk around the lake with me.

Toward the end of his life, I visited him in the hospital. His every move required the assistance of a nurse. He couldn't speak; however, his expressive eyes said, *This is where I don't want to be.* Later, I watched him quietly die. Surrounded by his family and friends, he was a man at peace. In contrast, other patients spent their "cancer time," being dominated by anger. *Bob taught me a lot about living and dying.*

At Christmas, because of the good fortune of our business, we had the opportunity to donate items from the store to the women's shelter in our community. Usually these products were scarfs and sweaters. One of the most poignant moments for me occurred when a woman approached the counter with tears in her eyes, carrying a small item that she wanted to purchase. "May I help you?" I asked.

"I—I came to thank you. Last year, when I was at the shelter, I received a present from your store. It made a big difference!"

As she left, I thought about the items I often gave to customers and friends. *It didn't do much for the bottom line of the store, but it did give me a great amount of satisfaction.* I received more than the recipient. Yes, through the years of Smedley's British Imports, my sense of contentment and peace continued to grow. I sold the business in 1990, following through on my gut feeling that it was time to begin simplifying my commitments. Throughout my life I have trusted my God-given instincts to guide my decisions.

Months later, one of our suppliers from Scotland who shipped handknit Aran sweaters to us, told me that the reason I had survived so long with leukemia was a result of the medicinal properties of the wool I handled every day. *Maybe my survival was just luck, or maybe it was a reflection of the guided steps I had taken for myself in my life.* All through this period I continued my conversations with God, asking for His direction.

When I was diagnosed with leukemia in August 1983, Chris was eight years old, Karen was ten, and Scott was thirteen. Each viewed my prognosis with differing levels of understanding. As each grew to understand my situation, they responded to me and my disease differently. Chris, the youngest, needed my physical touch. If I were lying on the floor or sitting on the couch, he wanted to be near me. Karen didn't want to hear any conversations regarding my illness. She avoided every mention of my leukemia. She did not want to accept the fact that her father might die at any time. Scott, the oldest, would verbalize his feelings. Once, as we were traveling together to a swimming meet in which he competed, we discussed the uncertainty of my future. I ended the conversation by saying, "Whatever happens to me, I will always be with you." He understood.

I felt I had to prepare the children to live a life without me. It was important to me that they learn the values and ethics that I believe are crucial for a good life. When an individual lives as good a life as possible, I believe earthly happiness follows. I was always conscious not to dwell on my illness while, at the same time, instilling in my children an understanding of the beauties in each day of our lives.

It is very difficult to describe the emotions Iva and I were feeling as wife and husband. I think each of us buried certain emotions for self-protection. We were preparing for what we were told was the "predictable" outcome. Preparing Iva and the kids for when I wasn't there meant that each of their lives had to be in order. Because I had previously handled all the finances of our household, I began shifting these responsibilities to Iva. She understood and began asking more questions about the family financial obligations. I watched her grow more independent and more self-assured of her abilities. It was comforting to know that she was strong enough to successfully guide the children's lives as well as her own.

All through this period, as I gained a greater appreciation for everything in this world, I would occasionally get what I called, "a rush of life," a high level of exhilaration and excitement about being alive. It was a sensation that is difficult to describe! It is something akin to the excitement I felt when, as a child, I would run down the stairs at Christmas time and see the presents under the tree. Another example is the triumph and feeling I enjoyed as a teenager, when I competed and won in sports.

During this period, the level of my meditation began to deepen. I could only achieve this deep level in two settings. As strange as it may sound, the first was sitting on the floor of my shower, usually with a wash cloth on my head, as the water soaked my body and blotted out the noise of the world. There was something hypnotic about the sound of the water as it hit me. The other setting I found conducive to meditation was sitting in the sand as the ocean surf pounded the beach. Accompanied by our children, and with our friends

Karen and Chris and Kathy and George and their children, these trips to the shore were times of great relaxation and joy. The results of the meditation at the ocean were much better than those achieved in the shower. This fact became evident to me in 1990 when, after a very pleasant week at Fenwick Island, New Jersey, I returned to Greensburg to find that my white blood count, although still above normal, had dropped by 10,000 from the previous week.

My meditation always began with a moment of relaxation and deep breathing. As my body began to relax, I visioned my spirit falling into this black emptiness within myself. When I achieved a sense of floating within my body, I would then concentrate on the specific parts of my body. I would think of words such as stability, equilibrium, and control, while visualizing the cells growing in my bone marrow, then holding them back—not releasing them into my blood stream—until they had matured. When visualizing certain bodily organs, I always thought "strong."

At one point, when I was having pains in my left side, it felt as if someone had stuck a knife into me. When my doctor examined me, he felt herniated tips or protusions on my spleen and suspected that my pains were a result of spleen infarctions. As he was preparing orders for a list of tests, I asked him if we could postpone the tests to see if I could first bring about a decrease in the pains myself. By this time, Dr. Dameshek, my hematologist, began to realize that maybe I did have some influence over my disease during my meditation and visualization sessions.

Following the visit, while meditating, I pictured two hands holding my spleen, relaxing it, caressing it, and "loving it." The next week, when I returned to my doctor, the pains had ceased and his examination failed to reveal any herniated tips. I never had a problem with my spleen again throughout the course of my illness.

During these years, as one goal was met, another one was

set. In 1987, when Scott graduated from high school and left to attend Virginia Tech, Iva also graduated with a degree in nursing and began working as a registered nurse in an oncology unit in a nearby hospital. At the time I was first diagnosed with leukemia, Iva was taking part-time college courses with the intention of becoming a social worker. My prognosis placed a sense of urgency on her plans. She felt that she must prepare for a career since she would probably be supporting three children by herself in the near future. The switch in majors gave her a difficult time with chemistry. She would lean her book against my back as she studied in bed each evening. The night of her graduation, I joked with her chemistry instructor that I had a permanent indentation in my back from the corner of her chemistry book. I was, and am, so very proud of my wife. She is a beautiful person in every way.

While working at the hospital, Iva would often return home crying because of the death of one of her patients. I knew what was happening. "Perhaps, you should transfer to a floor without cancer patients," I said gently.

She was emphatic with her answer. "No, that's not the answer. I am right where God wants me. Because of our situation I have special understanding and empathy for what the families are going through."

There were times when it seemed as if all of our lives were turned totally upside down by my illness; however, we always landed on our feet. Each family member took on additional and different roles. As we became stronger individuals and much closer as a family unit, it was evident that much good had come of the bad we had experienced.

In 1990, as I approached the seventh anniversary of hearing that dreaded diagnosis, my belief in the ability of the mind to help the body fight the progression of the leukemia continued to be strengthened by my successes. The love I had for my family, and their love and support in return, had given me additional strength to ward off the usual progression of the disease. I continued to thank God for His unending guidance which unfailingly boosted my faith and optimism so that I could continue to fight this battle and win.

CHAPTER III

You Need a Transplant

In August 1991, eight years after the initial diagnosis of leukemia and almost two years after my last bone marrow biopsy, I consented to be tested again. My reluctance to have a repeat biopsy was diminished by Iva's persuasion, and also signals from my own body. I had the feeling that something had changed. When you become as closely attuned to your body as I had become, the smallest changes are easily recognized.

I was not surprised when I heard the results the following month. The disease had moved into the accelerated phase. I was told that a patient may remain in the accelerated phase for a period of time ranging from two to eighteen months. This is then followed by the crisis stage of the disease—the blast stage—when a bone marrow transplant has little chance of success.

Dr. Dameshek, who had been my physician throughout the course of my illness, recommended that we start the process of looking for a potential donor. Because of our proximity to the University of Pittsburgh Medical Center and my former association with the facility, we initially began our donor search there. During the fall of 1991, the human leukocyte antigen (HLA) typing of more than 500,000 potential donors in the National Bone Marrow Registry was reviewed for a suitable match. None was found.

In October, my son Scott, who was in a Master's Degree program in biology at Virginia Tech in Blacksburg, Virginia, invited me to take a trip with him to the eastern shore of that state. We were going to collect soil specimens along the Chesapeake Bay to be analyzed for his thesis project. Our specimens were collected near farm fields, various distances from the Bay, in an effort to determine the extent that fertilizers being used in the surrounding area were ending up in the Bay. In truth I think his invitation was more intended to give us the opportunity to share some time together and for me to enjoy the beauty of nature as we canoed along the eastern shore. It was also a time that I could forget about the decisions and possibilities that lay ahead of me.

Scott's days had been filled with his research and his close friends, but generally he talked very little about the women in his life. On this trip, however, he talked a great deal about a young lady he had just met a few weeks earlier. He also wanted me to have dinner with the two of them when we returned to Blacksburg. With this preparation, I was not surprised when they announced their engagement a couple of months later. As I toasted Scott and Danielle at their engagement party, I said, "Watching the two of you together reminds me of when I fell in love with Scott's mother twenty-four years ago." As they planned their wedding for May 1992, I made a commitment to myself to be at the happy event.

In the hope of retarding the onset of the blast stage crisis of my illness, with my doctors orders, I began receiving daily interferon injections. This was in October of 1991. I was blessed that Iva could give me the injections. We would rotate the injection site between my arms and my legs. Initially, the interferon treatments brought on chills, fever, and fatigue; however, after a few days, the side effects subsided, leaving me feeling continually tired. The interferon therapy decreased my white blood cell count and, I believe, slowed the progression of the disease.

By January 1992, five months later, my doctors had not found a suitable donor. Iva and I decided to fly to Seattle, Washington to get a second opinion at the Fred Hutchinson Cancer Research Center, known colloquially as the "Hutch." The physician who performed the consult was Dr. C.D. Buckner; I liked him immediately. He gave me a sense of confidence that if I were going to have a transplant, this was the place to have it done. My confidence in the Hutch was strengthened when Iva and I toured the facility.

During this visit I asked Dr. Buckner what the possibility was of me having a successful transplant. He responded that based on the historical data of other patients in my stage of the disease, I had a thirty-five percent chance of surviving the transplant. When I expressed my disappointment with that number, he immediately helped me put the situation into proper perspective. He said that if someone had told me in 1983 that I had only a five percent chance of sitting in his office in Seattle in 1992, I would have felt an even greater disappointment. But, in reality, that was what I had done; I had lived into the last five percent of the survival curve. Although he couldn't predict my outcome, he was confident about my success based on my previous history. His comments and optimism were very encouraging to me.

The recommendation of the physicians at the Hutch was that Scott, my oldest son, should be my donor. As part of the donor search, my mother and dad, brother and sister, Iva, and all of our children had been HLA tested. Scott and Karen were identified as providing me with the closest match. Scott was chosen as the better of the two candidates due to his gender.

Because he had the genes and chromosomes of my wife Iva, he wasn't a perfect HLA match. The donation of his bone marrow to me was called a mismatch transplant. Interestingly, Scott's bone marrow was a closer match to mine than either that of my brother or sister. This was due, we learned, to the similarity that existed between the typing of my bone marrow and Iva's.

I was also told at the Hutch that I should have the transplant just as soon as it could be scheduled. *Time was running out for me!* I had been in the accelerated phase of my disease for at least six months. Scott and Danielle's wedding had been planned for May 16 which was four months away. When I returned home, I called the Director of the Hematology Laboratory at UPMC who had read my bone marrow biopsies since I was first diagnosed with leukemia in 1983. I asked him if, in his opinion, I could wait four months for my transplant so that I could attend my son's wedding. His answer was no; he recommended that I travel to Seattle as soon as they had an opening for me.

As I thought about the aspects of my life that had kept me alive during the previous nine years, I realized that I had lived for just such important events as Danielle and Scott's wedding. I wasn't going to change that thinking now. I called the people in Seattle, who by this time had scheduled my arrival for the first of April. Explaining my reason, I requested that the date be moved to the end of May. Hutch responded by writing my physician a letter which said that I was being optimistic that my disease would remain stable in the accelerated phase and that I should not postpone the transplant. After telling me this, my doctor simply said, "The decision is yours."

My decision had been made; I would attend my son's wedding!

Once the date was set for our departure—ten days after the wedding—I began the final preparations for the fight of my life. I had five months to galvanize all my resources, committing myself to prepare my body and mind as best I could for the unknown ordeal that lay ahead. Although I had been exercising three days a week for more than a year at the Aerobic Center in Greensburg, the sessions now became more intense. My goal was to get my body in the best possible shape prior to the transplant. During my exercise program of free weights and strengthening machines, I strived to put on additional muscle. I knew if I were bed ridden for a very long time, my muscle tissue would soon be lost. During each exercise, when I was reaching my peak of exertion, I would think, *One more repetition for Iva, one more for each of the children, or, this one is for Seattle.* Through the course of my interferon injections, my commitment to exercise never waned. As I began to see the results of my training program, I began to work even harder. I thought, *As I'm increasing my strength, each additional repetition is going to help me to return from Seattle.* I felt that the stronger I was going into the transplant, the stronger I would be coming out of it. I didn't realize at the time, however, how instrumental this exercise program would be in helping me survive the transplant.

My mental preparation for the transplant received equal importance. My meditations took on the words *peace, calm,* and *contentment.* Visual images began to be imprinted in my mind. I would walk around our yard or our pond, trying to observe as much as I could, close my eyes and mentally perform a review of what I had seen. I also did this with my family and friends, probably irritating them with my staring. I wanted to imprint these images in my mind, for I suspected there would be a time when my sensory stimulation would come solely from my mind. I began to tape some of my favorite music to be played continuously while I was in the Hutch. My thoughts were that the recovery process was going to be a mental journey, taking me back from any complications following the transplant. Though my body was weakened, I wanted my mind active and strong. I was striving to create the environment in my patient room that would be conducive for that journey. Without realizing it at the time, I was preparing my plan of survival.

At the wedding, I told my cousins Lee and Larry that I felt my recovery was going to be a mental journey and I felt sure that they and many other family members and friends would join me on this journey back to health. Eleven years earlier, Larry had undergone a kidney transplant. He understood my need for preparation.

Without consulting my physician, I had decided to stop the interferon injections one week prior to the wedding and then resume the injections immediately afterwards. This was a personal decision; however, I would not recommend that other patients stop any medication without their doctor's approval. I was determined to have the energy to dance and to enjoy every aspect of this family celebration.

As I sat in the historic church in Port Tobacco, Maryland and watched Scott and Danielle exchange wedding vows, I realized my preparations were now complete. I could leave for Seattle in ten days, knowing I was ready for whatever lay ahead of me. My emotions were overwhelming. Rob, one of the ushers in the wedding, referred to me the rest of the evening as, "Mr. Waterworks" because of my copious tears of joy. My satisfaction with my life, and the peace and contentment I felt came to a peak. Having done everything physically and mentally possible to prepare for the transplant, I acknowledged that my fate was now in God's hands.

I experienced one of my "rushes of life"—one of great happiness and joy while sitting in the church pew with Iva. As we listened to the beautiful violin music being played by Scott's friend Dave, who plays in the Audubon Quartet, I made a final pre-transplant commitment. My thoughts were prayer-like, *I want my grandchildren to know their grandfather based on experiences with me rather than from someone telling them about me.*

The wedding reception was beautiful. Chris, in his unique

way, expressed the love shared by our family and his love for his brother in his toast to Scott and Danielle. Iva and I joined Scott and Danielle during the wedding dance and, when I held Iva in my arms, I realized how blessed I had been. "I love you," I whispered. With my eyes I thanked her for sharing her life with me.

For me the highlight of the reception was watching Scott, and Chris and Scott's best man, Seth Miller, perform a dance routine. When I looked at Karen and then watched the two boys on the dance floor, I realized I had raised children who shared my love of life and were comfortable expressing their love for each other. Each of them carried a sense of goodness into every part of their lives. I was a very proud parent.

As my daughter Karen and I danced during the reception, she placed her head on my shoulder and began to cry. Her emotions, and the faces of friends and family in the room watching us, reminded me of the struggle that lay ahead.

During the last few months before my transplant, I had visited many of my former colleagues and friends. As one friend put it, I was saying my good-byes. At the end of this process, I had one more person I wanted to visit before I left for Seattle. If there ever was a living definition of a gentleman, it was Dwight. He was a retired chairman of a college Education Department who epitomized the personal characteristics that many of us strive to achieve. At the time of my visit, Dwight was suffering from prostate cancer that had spread to other organs of his body. He had been bed ridden for months. Often, after a visit with Dwight, my eyes would swell with tears as I left his house. He would never complain about his situation, but continually felt concern about the welfare of others. He gave of himself to his community, his church, his family, and his friends. For me, he was a powerful inspiration.

I think I had postponed my pre-Seattle visit to Dwight because I knew how difficult it was going to be for both of us. I told him that he was going to be the first person I would visit when I returned to Pennsylvania. I realized at the time that, due to his deteriorating condition, he might not survive the four months I'd be away. As I walked to the door to leave, Dwight called out, "If I am not here when you return, Jack, I'll save a seat in my pew for you." He died three weeks before I returned from Seattle. I often think of Dwight and his courage. He was a man of great integrity and strength.

David Clement, our pastor, had asked me what he and the congregation of the church could do for me prior to my leaving for Seattle with Iva and my son Scott. My only request was to have a healing service on the Sunday before we were to leave. Sitting in the church that Sunday, and standing before the altar during the Lutheran healing service, solidified and strengthened my resolve. When the pastor placed his hand on my forehead to bless me, the final component of my preparation was complete. I was now spiritually, as well as emotionally and physically, prepared.

Following the church service, the Mursches, Townes, and Smedleys had lunch together. The time we spent in the restaurant that day was so very symbolic of our friendship through the years. We laughed and we cried but, most of all, we gave each other support.

All that was left for me to do now was pack for Seattle.

CHAPTER IV

Summer in Seattle

Pre-transplant

On May 26, 1992, Iva and I left our home in Pennsylvania for the Fred Hutchinson Cancer Research Center in Seattle, Washington. Our son Scott had flown from Virginia to meet us in Pittsburgh, and from there we continued on our journey to the Northwest. Scott's wife Danielle had remained in Virginia, planning to fly to Seattle prior to the transplant. Scott and Danielle had returned from their honeymoon only two days earlier, and now Scott was leaving his new bride to donate bone marrow for his father's transplant. The strength of these newlyweds, now apart, in the earliest stages of their marriage, was remarkable. As Scott said, "The remainder of our lives should be smooth sailing after this."

Prior to leaving, Iva and I had decided to maintain journals during our time in Seattle. Extracts from these journals, shown in the indented text, are the best reflection of our emotions and state of mind during our stay. Often, however, we were physically too tired or too busy to document the day's events, and, for Iva, the pressures and the desire to remain strong for her family—especially for me—often precluded her express-ing her true emotions. We have, therefore, added some com-ments of the day's events following each journal entry.

MAY 26, 1992—TUESDAY

(IVA) Arrived in Seattle at 3:20 PM, weather sunny and 62 degrees—a good omen. The departure from Pittsburgh was emotional. George and Kathy took us to the airport where we met Scott who had flown from Roanoke, Va. We are fortunate to have George and Kathy as friends. They have been so sup-portive, as have been so many other people over the last few months. We took a taxi from the airport in Seattle to the First Hill Apartments where we will be staying. The reality is starting to set in; we have started on the road to Jack's new beginning.

It was a tearful good-bye at the airport with George and Kathy. Kathy gave me a book by one of my favorite authors. We tried to keep things light, but it was still an emotional time for all.

The hardest part of that day was leaving our home and our children Karen and Chris. My heart was so sad thinking of them at home, being on their own and trying to continue their daily routine—Karen going to work each day and Chris off to high school. I kept thinking how much I would miss them and the "mother" part of me wanted to be there with them to help them through what was to come. Praying that they would be okay, I acknowledged that they were both strong individu-als.

I felt so many emotions as I walked through each room of our home before we left. I kept thinking. *When will we come home again and will Jack be coming home with me?* I knew I would miss the comfort and familiarity of being in our home and having our friends nearby. This was probably the hardest thing I would ever have to do. I knew I would miss work and all the people there who gave me so much support. Although, I felt as if I were being pulled in many directions, my first priority was to help Jack get through the transplant. Whatever that would take, I would do it.

As Jack and I were flying to Seattle I thought about the events that had brought us to this point. I remembered the day when his diagnosis was confirmed by a second opinion; I felt as if everything stopped and then started again, but in slow motion. I'd wondered, *How must Jack be feeling?* I couldn't believe this was happening to him—to us—to our family. He was young, just thirty seven, and we had so much to do in our lives. Our children needed a father. *How could we tell them what was happening?*

Leukemia! *How I hated the word!* As a young child, I had learned that it was a very frightening word . . . I had been named after my grandmother, and her husband—my grandfather—had died from leukemia. He had been considerably older and only lived a few months after he was diagnosed. How ironic that my husband also had leukemia. *Would he die too?* I didn't even want to say the word leukemia. *But, if I'm frightened,* I thought, *how must our children feel?* I remember those first few nights following the meeting with his doctor. Sleepless nights tossing and turning. Jack and I would sit up in bed most of the time, talking about how we felt and what might happen. Those first few weeks were the hardest. If we had not had the love and support from our family and friends, it would have been even more difficult.

(**JACK**) Well we are here! Leaving home was not as difficult as I thought. Although somewhat stunned, I have been preparing for this day for so long, I am relieved that the time is finally here. I feel good about what is going to happen. It is going to take Iva and the kids awhile to adjust to our situation. I am trying to keep things light. Physically, I am feeling pretty good. I am definitely apprehensive, but ready to begin my journey.

Leaving for Seattle was the final step in the process I had begun months before. I had prepared myself mentally and physically as best I could. Now it was time. I was ready.

As I climbed the ramp to enter the plane, I looked back at Kathy and George. I will never forget the look on their faces. It was one of fear, but also hope.

MAY 27, 1992—WEDNESDAY

(IVA) Awake at 4:30 AM, back to sleep and awake at 6:00 AM. We went down to the waterfront early in the morning. Purchased fresh fruits, vegetables, and Alaskan shrimp which Scott picked out and prepared for dinner (they were delicious). Cooking has become a hobby for Scott and he enjoys it thoroughly. We also purchased French bread still warm from the oven. We had an appointment at the clinic at 2:00 PM. Jack and Scott had blood drawn and Jack had a physical. We received more information and a schedule of tests. Scott has been great. It's been good to have him here with us. We are all adjusting.

Giving over control to the system began. Our lives were being regulated by Jack's scheduled tests and examinations. Our apartment was adequate. We had all the necessities: two bedrooms, bath, small living area, and small kitchenette with dining area. I added pictures of our family and always tried to

44

have fresh flowers so the apartment would feel like home. The view of the city was nice. Outside was a small courtyard with tables and chairs. There were flowers all around. There was a small room by the front desk in the lobby with books, puzzles, etc. There always seemed to be someone in there. People were very friendly. It seemed like a miniature United Nations in our building. There were so many people from other countries.

> **(JACK)** Had our first taste of the health care delivery system at the "Hutch" (blood drawn). White blood cells (WBC) down to 34,000 (normal range 5,000-11,000) and platelets 161,000 (normal range 150,000-300,000). I think my body is stabilizing for the transplant. I am working to create that stabilization. The adjustment to our new environment seems easy, like a natural progression. I will have a variety of tests tomorrow and a bone marrow biopsy on Friday. I still have no fear. Anxious to get on with the procedure. It is nice to see Iva and Scott enjoying each other so much.

Prior to leaving for Seattle, and during the time I was there, I never felt afraid. My sense of peace was a combination of my religious beliefs, my contentment with my life, and the fact that I had prepared myself to the limits of my capabilities. Often I would think, *This is the fight of my life and I am ready.*

MAY 28, 1992—THURSDAY

> **(IVA)** Our third day went well. We had a conference with Jack's physician. Sunny all day and a little rain this evening. Each day we are adjusting to the

45

time change a little more. Jack and Scott had chest x-rays. I was given a reference notebook and a number of other papers for bone marrow transplant patients. I started to carry a canvas bag to hold all of this information. It is becoming my constant companion.

Being a registered nurse, and also oncology certified, gave me an advantage in being able to adapt to the information and changes that were happening so quickly.

(JACK) Met with my the attending physician today. She told us all the things that could go wrong and possible complications. I realize, now, how little I know about what is going to happen to me. I feel sorry for Scott. I hate that he has to go through this, especially at this time in his life. I told Scott that I hope I don't have long-term complications from the transplant. I would rather not survive the procedure than to live a life plagued with health problems. Still fairly calm. Will have bone marrow biopsy tomorrow. I had, what I hope, was my last shot of interferon last night. Will start exercising Sunday at Seattle University. I need to exercise. Iva is relaxed tonight; her shoulders and neck have been bothering her (I guess it is the stress). It's difficult to describe our reactions to the changes that are taking place in our lives. Really concentrating on keeping my body and mind in equilibrium.

At this point I began to realize why, when I joked that the transplant was going to be "Daddy's big adventure," that Iva kept such a stern face. She knew what ordeal lay ahead of me.

46

MAY 29, 1992—FRIDAY

(IVA) Another beautiful day. We went to the clinic. Jack and Scott had blood drawn and EKG'S. Jack had a bone marrow biopsy and Scott had a physical. Met with the dietitian and she explained nutritional requirements and hyperalimentation with which I was already familiar. Scott and I went grocery shopping and Scott cooked dinner. After dinner, Jack and I walked over to the Seattle University gym. Telephoned Chris tonight; the Mursches were there along with my mother and father. Sounds as if they are doing okay.

It was interesting to see the nurses doing the bone marrow biopsies; I was accustomed to a doctor performing this procedure.

Seattle was a nice city. The mountains were very inspiring. Looking out over Elliott Bay and the Olympic Mountains had a very calming effect. I enjoyed that view during our many visits to the outpatient clinic and I would always marvel at the beauty.

(JACK) Met a nice couple from Indiana today: Scott and Jeanne Dudley. He also has CML. I had my bone marrow biopsy today and it wasn't painful. During the procedure I was mentally walking around our pond. We are going to Mt. Rainier tomorrow; looking forward to being out in nature. I feel sad for Scott and Iva. This is difficult for both of them.

Iva told me later that at one point during the bone marrow biopsy, I was asked if I felt okay. When I didn't respond, the nurse became alarmed. Iva told her not to worry, that my body was there, but my mind was somewhere else.

The day we met the Dudleys, we were originally sitting at opposite ends of the clinic. I think all of us were looking a little tired from our experiences in Seattle. I approached Scott and asked him if he too were preparing for a transplant. It was comforting to share and hear the feelings of someone else about to take the same journey.

MAY 30, 1992—SATURDAY

(IVA) The weather is really cooperating. We rented a car and drove to Mt. Rainier. It is beautiful scenery with snow capped mountains. Scott, our son, wasn't feeling well, but he still went with us. I think he wants to spend as much time with us as possible. I know he misses Danielle.

The road leading up the mountain was not my idea of fun. I was a little anxious on all those curves. We had lunch at Paradise Lodge near the top. Snow was all around. We all enjoyed the day.

(JACK) Great day! Mt. Rainier was magnificent. As beautiful a place as I have ever seen. Short entry today; we drove 230 miles and I'm tired.

Every chance I had, I found a way to enjoy the creations of God, for I knew my physical isolation would soon begin. I continued to create images in my mind so that I would never feel mental iolation.

48

MAY 31, 1992—SUNDAY

(IVA) Up at 6:00 AM. Scott's flight left at 8:15 AM. Also went to Pike Street Market and purchased fruits, vegetables, and fresh flowers Met a couple from Pennsylvania; the husband was back for his one-year checkup. He is thirty-six and also had CML and is doing very well. After they left, Jack and I walked around the block. I started reading a new book.

Reading was an escape for me. It also helped me pass many hours in Seattle. I made frequent trips to the book store. Shopping at the Pike Street Market was a wonderful experience. I loved looking at all the fresh flowers and smelling the mixture of fresh baked bread, fruits, vegetables and the fresh sea air from Elliott Bay.

(JACK) Long day. We took Scott to the airport and then stopped at the University of Washington Arboretum. Saw many Canadian geese. Had a visit with a Pennsylvania man who had a transplant last year. It is very difficult for me to hear the experiences of other people when I am at the beginning of that same road. In some ways, it is better not to know as much in the beginning. I guess I can't know what I'll experience. It is depressing to learn that I won't be able to do any gardening for a year after the transplant, for fear of being exposed to various bacteria and fungus in the soil.

Following the completion of Scott's pre-donor tests and the uncertainty of when I would enter the hospital, we thought it best if he returned home to Danielle. We would notify him when we knew more about my situation.

JUNE 1, 1992—MONDAY

(IVA) Jack had blood drawn and then we had
breakfast at Swedish Hospital cafeteria. Met with a
social worker who will assign a volunteer to help us
while we are in Seattle. Tonight Jack watched a hockey
game while I read.

Athough I had found the laundry room and started getting
into a routine, I still missed our home and our life there. Meeting more families helped ease the feeling of loneliness. Our
volunteers, Cindy and Bob, helped ease the transition to our
new home in Seattle. They were wonderful. When I needed
to get away to replenish my emotional strength, Bob would
find a great place for lunch or a nice restaurant with excellent
desserts. He also told us many interesting stories about the
city of Seattle.

(JACK) Not much to write about. Blood drawn
and a visit to social service. I am very anxious to
begin. Probably will not feel that way once the process starts. Being around all these patients and their
families, you hear so many horror stories. It seems as
if every patient had a crisis and almost died! I hope
I'm strong enough to survive mine. *I wonder what it
will be?*

JUNE 2, 1992—TUESDAY

(IVA) Karen called today. Sounds as though she's
doing well. Jack had a pulmonary function test, arte-
rial blood gases, and an oral exam. Went to Pioneer
Square and had lunch. Ate dinner with the Dudleys
at McCormick's Fish House and bar.

Little did I know at this point what a close relationship Jeanne and I would have as the weeks passed. There are many people that you meet and pass by, but Jeanne and Scott Dudley have left a permanent imprint in our hearts. I will never forget the time we shared during that summer. I cannot imagine having lived through those four months without Jeanne's support and companionship.

The friendship that the Dudleys and Smedleys developed in those four months in Seattle will last a lifetime.

> **(JACK)** Had a variety of tests done today. I'm tired tonight.

In many ways, we and the Dudleys were acting as though we were on vacation in the Northwest. We did a great deal of sight-seeing and ate at some wonderful restaurants. I gained five pounds during this three week period before I entered the Hutch. Scott Dudley and I decided that we were not going to sit around our apartments and worry about what the future would hold for us. We decided that we were definitely going to enjoy ourselves before we entered the Hutch.

JUNE 3, 1992—WEDNESDAY

> **(IVA)** Today we went by ferry to Winslow on Bainbridge Island with Jeanne and Scott Dudley. We walked around the town and looked in all the quaint shops. Had lunch at a little restaurant by the water. On our return to Seattle we saw Jeff Bridges filming a scene for the movie, called the "Vanishing," which is to be released next summer.

I have since seen the movie and enjoyed seeing all the places that I had become so familiar with while in Seattle. This day was another of many happy memories from our time in Seattle. As I took pictures of Jeff Bridges, Jeanne kept pushing me out into the area of the street where they were filming. She wanted me to get a close up. Jack and Scott were laughing at us. They said we were acting like a couple of teenagers.

JUNE 4, 1992—THURDAY

(IVA) The clinic called with news that Jack's liver function tests were elevated. We went to the clinic where Jack had an exam by a GI specialist. Later we had breakfast with the Dudleys. They tried to boost our spirits. It is good we met them. It has been nice to have someone with whom to discuss the events of the past week. Jack went to exercise in the afternoon at Seattle University and I took the van to the grocery store. We called Dr. Dameshek in Pittsburgh to let him know what was going on. His closing remark was, "I love you guys."

The "van" was the transportation vehicle provided by First Hill Apartments where we were staying. Gary was the van's full time driver; Norm (a volunteer) drove once a week. They were great! There were scheduled trips to the grocery store and continual daily trips back and forth from the apartments to the Hutch and outpatient clinic.

(JACK) Where do I begin? Received a call this morning that my liver function tests were elevated and that I was scheduled to see a GI physician immediately. Some components of the test were extremely high. Based on the tests results, I would have a 40%

chance of getting venous occlusive disease (VOD) following the transplant. My immediate reaction was that the VOD risk added to the risk of the transplant was just too much to surmount, but I eventually got over this feeling.

I called Dr. Dameshek to get the results of my liver function tests from March 4. They were normal. His reaction was the same as mine. Received a call tonight scheduling a sonogram and CT scan for tomorrow afternoon. Will have a liver function test again tomorrow morning. I believe they are looking for an obstruction. If they find one, I think the game is over and I will return home. The next few days will probably be the most intense in my life. My life truly is in God's hands.

"Veno-occlusive disease (VOD) is a disease of the liver that occurs in many bone marrow transplant (BMT) patients in the first few weeks post transplant. It can range in severity from very mild to serious. It is thought to be caused primarily by chemotherapy and radiation.

<u>Patient reference manual, Fred Hutchinson Cancer Research Center.</u>

Through the years, the patient-doctor relationship between Dr. Dameshek (PUH physician) and myself became a partnership. Each new decision regarding my care was thoroughly discussed, with the two of us deciding on the proper course of treatment. I will always be grateful for his acceptance of my desire to direct my own care.

53

JUNE 5, 1992-FRIDAY

(IVA) Today is my mom and dad's forty-fourth anniversary. Jack's creatinine was slightly elevated, so they wouldn't do the CT scan. Three people at the clinic tried to start an IV for Jack for hydration, but were not successful. Will try to do the scan again on Monday. They gave him instuctions to drink at least two liters of fluid a day over the weekend. Jack had a nap and we had a quiet evening.

(JACK) Another eventful day. Received a call this morning that my kidney functions were elevated and I should come to the clinic as soon as possible to receive hydration. After having two nurses try to insert the IV in each of my arms without success, I became very frustrated and requested that I talk to my physician before we proceeded. My physician explained that I was receiving the hydration because they suspected the interferon injections had caused the elevation in the liver functions tests, and that the antibiotic I was taking had caused the high kidney functions levels. I consented to have a third person (a phlebotomist) attempt to start the IV. He also failed. I then suggested that I drink a lot of water over the weekend and we try again Monday. The nurse gave me an estimate of the amount of the fluids I needed to drink. The insertion of the Hickman catheter was also postponed. Very frustrating day. I was close to saying enough, but I realize this is my only hope and I must give it my best.

"Hickman line- a large flexible tube inserted into the entrance of the heart through a major vein in the chest. It is used to draw blood specimens and infuse fluids,

54

parenteral nutrition and medications."

Patient reference manual, Fred Hutchinson Cancer Research Center.

JUNE 6, 1992—SATURDAY

(**IVA**) Jack had blood drawn early. Went on a day trip with the Dudleys to Bainbridge Island and Olympic National Park. The mountains are beautiful. We saw a herd of deer near the top of the mountain. We were able to walk very close to them.

Jeanne and I threw snowballs at Scott and Jack as we walked around the lookout on Hurricane Ridge in the Park. The importance of these happy times together prior to the transplant, in many ways, set the stage for both Scott and Jack's successful transplants.

These were periods in which we could relax and forget what lay ahead of us. For Scott and Jack this was the time they began the commitment to pull each other through their transplants. It was appropriate that they would enter the hospital the same day and receive their transplants within hours of each other.

JUNE 7, 1992—SUNDAY

(**IVA**) This certainly was a memorable day. Jack had blood drawn again early at the clinic and then we set off to Vancouver with the Dudleys. Visited Van

Deusen gardens and Granville Island. Following dinner, we started back to Seattle. The trip back turned
out to be a bit more exciting than the trip up. We
were stopped by the police (six cars in all). They
thought we were driving a stolen car! Our rental car
had previously been stolen and recovered but the rental
agency had failed to notify the authorities. Thus, it
was still on the list of stolen vehicles. It was a very
frightening experience. The police officers even
pulled their guns and had us hold our hands up! It
took us a while to get the situation resolved but, by
the time we arrived back in Seattle, we were able to
laugh about the incident.

(JACK) Visited Vancouver today. Beautiful city
in front of a ridge of mountains. Toured a botanical
garden. I lay down on a bench by a Scottish shelter in
the gardens and closed my eyes and listened to the
goslings in a nearby pond. What a relaxing place! I
visualized my body accepting and welcoming my son
Scott's bone marrow. Got some ideas for our pond at
home. I miss our yard and gardens, but I remember
them in my mind. Experienced a wild incident with
the police today.

As we were driving south from Vancouver, I noticed that a
police car had pulled in behind us. Then, in my rear view
mirror, I noticed a second patrol car with its lights flashing,
speeding toward us. When the patrolman saw us, he turned
the flashing lights off and pulled in behind the first patrol car.
Scott Dudley and I were in the front seat and Iva and Jeanne
were in the back seat.

When I told them about the police cars, they said I was
probably speeding, but I knew I hadn't exceeded the speed
limit. Jeanne suggested I pull off at the next exit and let the

police cars pass us. Based on later events, this would have been interpreted as an evasive tactic. I then saw two more patrol cars sitting in the median that immediately pulled out behind us as we passed. Then, with all the patrol cars' lights flashing, we were instructed to pull off the highway. By this time we were surrounded by six patrol cars on Interstate 5.

As I looked in the rearview mirror, I could see the police officers pulling out their revolvers as they approached the back of our car. Then, standing near the trunk of our car, they began shouting orders at us. Being on the side of a busy highway, we were unable to hear what they were shouting. Iva thought they were telling us to raise the trunk. I responded by saying that I had no idea where the trunk release button was located. Then Jeanne said they were telling us to raise our hands. We all promptly placed our hands on the ceiling of the car.

One police officer, revolver in hand, approached Scott's side of the car and asked him where we had obtained the car. Scott immediately pointed to me and said that I had rented the vehicle.

I was asked to produce the rental agreement. Escorted out of the car by two officers, I opened the trunk and got the rental agreement out of my coat. Upon examining my Pennsylvania driver's license, the officer wanted to know why I was in Washington. When I explained that I was going to receive a bone marrow transplant, and so was the other gentleman in the front seat, I received a very skeptical look. As Iva, Jeanne, and Scott all produced their driver's license, my wife approached one the officers and, in her most sincere voice, said, "I am a nurse and I wouldn't hurt anyone." After some discussion we learned the car we were driving was listed as a stolen vehicle. The first officer to follow us said he had checked the status of the car twice because, as he observed our behavior, we did not appear to be conducting ourselves as if we had committed any type of a crime. Subsequently, we learned the car had been stolen in Washington and retrieved in Chicago. When it was returned to Seattle, it was never removed from the official list of stolen vehicles. The end result of this incident was that both the Smedleys and Dudleys received a free rental car during our stay in Seattle.

JUNE 9, 1992—TUESDAY

(IVA) Indecision about the elevated liver functions. Met with GI specialists and Jack's attending physician. After much discussion and sole searching, we decided to go ahead with the transplant. Karen was upset when she called tonight. This is so difficult for everyone. I feel as if I'm being torn in several different directions.

It was probably good that Jack didn't know that he would experience all the problems and complications that he was told might occur after the transplant. I remember his saying at one point, "If I had known it was going to be like this, I would not have come to Seattle." But, after he recovered, his thoughts and feelings changed and he was glad he went through with the transplant. I remember how frustrated and helpless I felt, not being able to be with Karen and Chris at home, and also not able to give Jack assurance that everything would be okay.

(JACK) The roller coaster ride continues! At 3:00 PM we had our data review conference and met with three different physicians. Very depressing! Because of the type of match with my son, I have a five to ten percent chance of Scott's bone marrow rejecting my body. Also, because of my elevated liver functions, I have a forty percent chance of developing

58

venuous occlusive disease (VOD). I realize now the extent of my battle to survive this procedure. I must maintain an attitude of never giving up and the desire to succeed. I feel very committed. To return home without having the transplant is to return to certain death.

With the additional risks of VOD and rejection, I was told that my chance for a successful transplant decreased from thirty-five percent to between fifteen and twenty percent.

JUNE 10,1992—WEDNESDAY

(IVA) Spent most of the day at Swedish Hospital Day Surgery. Jack had a Hickman Line inserted without difficulty. Bob and Cindy, our volunteers, stopped by for a visit this evening.

Bob was a student at the University of Washington. His plans included medical school and he was a very warm and happy person. Bob and Cindy's preparation for volunteer work at the Hutch had included twenty-five hours of orientation and training. Cindy was also a student at the University of Washington, majoring in international finance. She was a very bright and caring young lady. They provided both practical and emotional support for us during our stay in Seattle.

(JACK) Had blood work this morning and then was sent to the outpatient surgery department for the insertion of the Hickman catheter. Scott Dudley was already there. He was scheduled before me. I have truly enjoyed his friendship. He and his wife Jeanne have been a pleasure. This would have been a tough week without them. Woke up in the recovery room with Scott Dudley laughing at me from the bed beside me. Seems natural to have these tubes sticking out of me. It is amazing how the mind can adjust.

Prior to the insertion of the catheter, I met with the anesthesiologist who was to describe the procedure. He informed me that I would endure great pain. Then he laughted and said "Mr. Dudley told me to scare you as much as I could." I then received the correct information concerning the insertion of the Hickman line Even though we were often dealing with very serious subjects, the Dudleys and Smedleys always found something to laugh about. I can not over empahsize the importance of this laughter. Although I tried to laugh at least once a day, I am sure there were many days when I failed in this goal.

JUNE 11, 1991—THURSDAY

(IVA) Our son Scott arrived today. Went to the Hutch with Jeanne for Hickman care class. Then had my blood drawn for CMV status and HIV test. This evening we went to Elliott's restaurant with the Dudley's and Scott. The waiting is getting very difficult. I wish Jack could get started with everything.

The pressure on family members is immense. During my training session on the care and cleaning of the Hickman line, a spouse of a pre-transplant patient stood up and explained that she couldn't handle this any more and walked out. I am not sure what became of her and her husband.

JUNE 12, 1992—FRIDAY

(IVA) Jack had blood drawn while I went to Puget Sound Blood Donation Center with our son Scott. He gave blood to be stored and given back to him after he donates his bone marrow. Rained most of the day.

Donating his blood for storage was another new experience for our son Scott. The Galiotto's, our friends and former neighbors in Greensburg, who were now living in Washington, came by that evening. We spent the hours reminiscing about the "old times" and things we had done together.

JUNE 13, 1992—SATURDAY

(IVA) The waiting is getting harder and harder each day. Spent most of the day cleaning and doing laundry. Karen and Chris arrive tomorrow!!

We found out later that the wait was a result of the time needed for approval of a protocol designed to help reduce the possibility of Scott's bone marrow rejecting Jack's body. The day after it was approved, Jack was admitted to the hospital.

JUNE 14, 1992—SUNDAY

(IVA) Sunny and cool. Karen and Chris arrived at noon. It was really good to see them. Chris was anxious for us to see the video he had made of our old home movies . He added appropriate music. We cried and laughed as we watched it after dinner. It is really good to have everyone together again. If only

Danielle could be here, our family would be complete.

(JACK) I guess I've been lackadaisical in completing my journal. Picked the kids up today. It was really great to see them. They seem to like this place. When Danielle arrives, I hope they can do some sight seeing. Scott Dudley and I should enter the hospital Tuesday. I hope we both do well. I am still at peace with my situation; I hope that continues. We have been here for almost three weeks and the time has gone fast. I am worried about the rejection of Scott's bone marrow. I will be so happy when Scott's bone marrow begins to grow in my body!

JUNE 15, 1992—MONDAY

(IVA) We all went to dinner at Ivar's on the waterfront with Jeanne and Scott Dudley and their daughter Robin. Was a nice evening.

That evening was a time of excitement and of anticipation of the days ahead. I was filled with a mixture of feelings: happiness and a sense of anxiety, and uncertainty as to what would be the outcome for us all. Throughout dinner and later, we took pictures of our families. We certainly didn't look like two families about to begin an ordeal.

(JACK) Tomorrow should be the day. Scott Dudley and I talked at dinner that we are anxious to get on with it. Probably, after it begins, we will be wishing we were back having dinner at Ivar's. As I looked around the table, I was so very proud of our children and gave most of the credit for that to Iva. During their younger years I spent most of my time

62

working. God give me strength to walk back from
the hell that I will endure.

CHAPTER V

Summer in Seattle

Transplant

I thought I was ready for what lay ahead of me, but never in my worst dreams could I have imagined what was to occur to my body during the next thirty-five days while hospitalized in the Hutch. Although I made a few entries in my journal following my admission, they are not readable ... even to myself. To depict the physical stress my body was under, Iva and I extracted information from my daily medical record during my hospitalization. This medical information is underlined and introduces each day. Iva's journal entries and comments continue in this chapter as they were presented in chapter IV. My recollection of events, thoughts, and feelings each day during my hospitalization are presented in italics.

JUNE 16, 1992—TUESDAY

(MEDICAL RECORDS) Patient and family supportive of each other, each handling situation in individual fashion. Family stayed through evening. Slight headache after lumbar puncture.

> **(IVA)** The call finally came that we have been waiting for: Jack is to be admitted to the Fred Hutchinson Cancer Research Center at noon. Lots of mixed emotions. Jack is ready! So am I. Scott is at the airport picking up Danielle. I think we have everything packed. Jack, Karen, Chris and I rode the van to the Hutch. Chris made a video of Jack's admission. At 2:00 PM we six Smedley's had a family conference with Jack's primary and attending physicians, nurse, and physician assistant. At 6:00 PM lumbar puncture was performed by the physician assistant. Following the procedure, Jack took a sterile bath and entered the laminar airflow room (LAF). With the assistance of his nurse, he took his LAF medicines and used his creams, powders, and ointments. The powders and creams were applied to various entrances to Jack's body. Preparation and entering LAF is like dressing for a "moon walk." Stayed with Jack till 11:00 PM and then returned to the apartment on the van.

The day Jack was admitted was one we had all been waiting for. It was a day of high emotion. I had thought I wanted the day to come but, when it did, I wasn't sure I wanted Jack to begin the treatment for the transplant. I wanted a guarantee that he would be okay, but I knew that was not possible.

It was helpful that Scott Dudley was admitted on the same day. I know the staff at the Hutch thought it was quite unusual that we were so connected to each other. It was as if we had checked into a hotel and we were now surveying each other's rooms! At the family conference, more information was given by the physicians and we asked a lot of questions.

(JACK'S RECOLLECTIONS) *During the lumbar*

puncture procedure, my mind was at home, standing by the pond listening to the waterfall and the birds singing. It is amazing to me that this technique can really minimize the pain and discomfort. The physician assistant had trouble in obtaining the spinal fluid. He told me to inform the next person performing the procedure to use a long needle and to point it upward. I expressed the desire that there would not be a "next time."

Scott Dudley's room is two rooms away from mine. As we prepared to enter our sterile rooms, I shook his hand and said, "See you when we get out." Very difficult to describe the emotions I felt at that time. In my room, on my wall writing board, were two telephone numbers: the Hutch kitchen and "Dud." The nurses on the unit told us this was the first time they ever had patients calling each other from their LAF rooms. Our close friendship actually caused great concern for the staff at the Hutch. They felt if one of us didn't survive, it was going to be very detrimental to the other.

JUNE 17, 1992—WEDNESDAY

(MEDICAL RECORDS) <u>Headache position-dependent much worse when standing up. Rash on arms and legs. Foley catheter inserted for continuous bladder irrigation.</u>

(IVA) Arrived at the Hutch around 9:00 PM. Gowned with the assistance of Jack's nurse and helped him with his bath, powders, and creams. I am spending the night since Jack is having problems with his IV (constantly beeping). Also, the caffeine (for his headache, a result of the lumbar puncture) is causing some excitability. Jeanne came in at midnight and wished me a happy birthday. I had forgotten that Thursday was my birthday.

I slept in a chair near Jack's bed because the infusion pump kept beeping all night. He was on the other side of a plastic partition that separated the outer room from the patient area. His IV pole and medications were on my side of the room with lines extending through the partition that were connected to his Hickman line. The plastic partition contained rubber sleeves and gloves which the nurses would use when they touched Jack or his infusion lines. I had to keep getting up all night and resetting the machine.

JUNE 18, 1992—THURSDAY

(MEDICAL RECORDS) Patient became quite nauseated, required multiple medications to control.
Patient taking very shallow breaths. He could not take deep breaths even with encouragement.

(IVA) During the night I slept for about 1-1/2 hours in a chair in Jack's room. Jack finally went to sleep around 4:00 AM. I went back to the apartment at 6:30 AM and took a hot bath and rested for about an hour. Went to breakfast with Scott and Danielle, then stopped by the hospital. Jack is sleeping. Went to a family support meeting and they surprised me with a birthday cake. Jack is not having a very good day. It's so difficult to see him like this. Spent all day at the hospital, then came back to the apartment for dinner. We had pizza and a birthday cake. Jack had given Scott pearl earrings to give to me. Scott and Danielle gave me a nice vase made in Seattle filled with fresh flowers from the market. I cried. Chris and

Karen gave me a card and birthday balloons. It is difficult to even think about a birthday when Jack feels so bad. I just wish I could do something to help him. We went back to see Jack after we finished dinner. Karen is staying with him tonight.

JUNE 19, 1992—FRIDAY

(Medical Records) Continued nausea and vomiting with chills. Rash, right shoulder. Temperature 102.9 F. Blood in urine. Chest x-ray performed.

(IVA) I went up to the hospital about 8:00 AM after Karen and I had breakfast. Jack is sleeping. He had a better night. He is still having nausea/vomiting, diarrhea and a fever. The Lutheran minister came by and conducted a communion service for all of us, which was very nice. I stayed until about 10:00 PM, when Chris picked me up. Jack is still having diarrhea (a result of the chemotherapy).

JUNE 20, 1992—SATURDAY

(Medical Records) Blood cultures drawn. Temperature 102.7 F. Patient anxious. Diarrhea.

(IVA) Karen leaves today. I really wish she could stay longer, but she must return to work. I know she is having a very difficult time thinking about Jack. I wish I could make it easier for her and everyone else. Jack had his first radiation treatment at 7:30 AM. He hasn't been able to eat. He is still having nausea and vomiting. Tried Jello, but he couldn't eat it. Karen said good-bye and Scott and Danielle took her to the airport. It was hard saying good-bye. I hope I can keep myself together through all of this.

Chris and I had lunch and then went back to sit with Jack. I went with him for his second radiation therapy. He must be so scared. I know I'm scared for him. This just doesn't seem real. Chris and I stayed at the hospital and then returned to the apartment to wash Jack's slippers and robe. Chris and Robin Dudley sat out in the sun and talked. I returned to the hospital when the clothes were dry. Jack is up and down and sleeping intermittently. He had just returned from radiation therapy; I know he is exhausted.

Karen called while we were doing Jack's bath. She had arrived home safely. We returned to the apartment at 9:30 PM. Chris is watching TV. I know he is thinking about the BMT because he asked some questions tonight and I tried to answer them as well as I could.

I'm so proud of our children and how well they were able to cope with the whole experience of the time before, during, and after the transplant. And I know it was not easy for Danielle to have just become a part of our family and been thrown into this situation She was very understanding and supportive. She has become our second daughter.

JUNE 21, 1992-SUNDAY

(MEDICAL RECORDS) <u>Vomiting continues, treated</u> <u>with medication.</u>

(IVA) Jack is still having nausea, vomiting, and diarrhea. He is sleeping most of the time with the aid of medication. Received platelets for the first time today.

"Platelets — a type of blood cell that helps your blood to clot"

 <u>Patient reference manual, Fred Hutchinson Cancer Research Center.</u>

JUNE 22, 1992—MONDAY

(MEDICAL RECORDS) <u>Patient's breath sounds intermittently coarse. Patient encouraged to use breath exercise device. Additional medication given for nausea with good results.</u>

(IVA) Jack's third day of radiation. An emotional day, as he talked about what he has been seeing during his radiation therapy. Jack will be getting two units of red blood cells today. I found out today that I am CMV+, so I cannot give platelets to Jack.

Jack was so frightened during this phase of the treatment. I never felt so helpless as I did during this time. Chris and I were both CMV+, Karen, Scott and Jack were CMV-, so Chris and I couldn't donate platelets to Jack. We were both very disappointed.

"CMV (cytomegalovirus) — a virus that can cause pneumonia or other infections in BMT patients"

Patient reference manual, Fred Hutchinson Cancer Research Center

(JACK'S RECOLLECTIONS) *I received eleven radiation treatments, each approximately twenty minutes in length. I am not sure of the reason, but at first I would sleep and have horrible nightmares, crying when I awoke. About half way through the eleven sessions, I finally succeeded in mentally leaving the room and visiting past pleasurable memories in my life. My nightmares and crying stopped.*

JUNE 23, 1992—TUESDAY

(MEDICAL RECORDS) Edema beginning on ankles. Diarrhea continues. Rash fading. Two units of red blood cells given.

(IVA) Jack has been at the Hutch one week today. He looks a little better. Has been on total parenteral nutrition since Friday. He finished radiation this afternoon. I helped him with his bath after radiation. His rash has receded, I read him the cards and notes that we had received during the week and he seemed to really enjoy it. Mom and Dad Smedley arrived this evening. Jack seems so much better. Chris dressed and went into the LAF with Jack this evening and they played cards and talked. All of us went out to

72

dinner tonight, except Chris who stayed at the apartment and had pizza with Jeanne and Robin. Following dinner, we went to the Hutch and stayed with Jack until 9:30 PM. Tomorrow is the big day. Scott is getting anxious. I got a card and wrote a note to him. It is hard to put everything into words that I feel. Karen called Jack today. I miss her and wish she could be here.

Many times throughout these four months in Seattle, I felt torn and pulled in various directions. It was very frustrating for me not to be able to be with Karen and Chris when they were at home and, at the same time, watching the torment that Jack was going through.

JUNE 24, 1992—WEDNESDAY

(MEDICAL RECORDS) Feet are still swollen. Nausea and occasional vomiting. Blood pressure elevated. Beginning mucositis. Pencil-sized [diameter] blood blisters on the inside of cheeks.

(IVA) This is the day! Scott went in to see Jack before going over to Swedish Hospital to be admitted to donate his bone marrow. Danielle and I went with him. Jack started receiving Scott's bone marrow about 2:20 PM. He had received platelets earlier. Scott and Danielle came over to the Hutch to see Jack this evening. Scott is sore but doing okay. I stayed with Jack till 11:00 PM. Now we wait.

Jack looked so ill. I remember thinking how difficult it was to see him this way. Jeanne and I were walking by the nursing station when we saw the bag containing the bone

73

marrow that Scott had donated lying on the counter. I had a strange feeling knowing it had just been taken from Scott and it would soon be given to Jack. Scott Dudley was to receive his marrow from a donor in England. We were all relieved when we heard the plane had arrived carrying his marrow. He received his marrow that same evening.

Early in Jack's hospitalization, due to his condition, it was very difficult to understand him when he was speaking. Scott Dudley told his wife, Jeanne, that he was getting very upset because he couldn't understand a word Jack was saying when he called him. As Scott Dudley became increasingly distraught when he heard of Jack's deteriorating condition, a notice was posted in the nursing station for the staff not to discuss Jack's condition with him.

"Mucositis - irritation and ulceration of the mouth caused by the side effects of chemotherapy and radiation. This can cause significant mouth pain and be a source of infection."

Patient reference manual, Fred Hutchinson Cancer Research Center.

(**Jack's Recollections**) *The amount of bone marrow extracted from the donor is determined by the weight of the recipient. In my case, Scott donated over a liter of marrow. It was extracted from the right and left posterior iliac crest. A needle was inserted in six sites multiple times to acquire the quantity of bone marrow needed. Scott's bone marrow was given to me through the IV line in my chest. The miraculous aspect of this procedure is the donor marrow travels through the blood stream to the recipient's bone marrow cavities where it hopefully will begin reproducing.*

JUNE 25, 1992—THURSDAY

(MEDICAL RECORDS) Patient's mouth and tongue becoming more painful. Breathing very shallow. Pain and toxicity consult ordered. Platelets given. Patient has nausea with dry heaves.

(IVA) Danielle and I went to Swedish Hospital about 8:30 AM to see Scott. He was discharged by 10:00 AM from the hospital. We then went over to see Jack who had a restless night. Very fidgety, up and down, can't concentrate on anything. They had given him Compazine for his nausea during the night. He started on Marinal (marijuana) for nausea. I had a conference with Jack's doctor concerning his medications and the possibility of breaking LAF. Took Scott and Danielle to the airport to catch their flight. Jack was given Cogentin and Ativan in late afternoon without any decrease in restlessness. I went to the apartment at 9:00 PM and returned about midnight. Around 1:00 AM he came out of LAF. I stayed until he went to sleep at 4:00 AM and then returned to the apartment. At 5:45 AM his nurse called me and said Jack was on oxygen via face mask and that his oxygen saturation level was only 82% (normal range: above 92%). I came back to the Hutch and they were doing a stat electrocardiogram, chest x-ray, and another pulse oxygen level. Chest x-ray showed fluid in the lungs. Electrocardiogram normal. Jack's physician and physician assistant went in early to see him. They reviewed everything and returned later. Jack is showing early signs of VOD and he is in fluid overload.

When a patient broke LAF, the nursing staff would remove the plastic partition that separated the patient area from the remainder of the room, thus destroying the sterile area that was created for the patient. I believe Jack's desire for freedom from LAF was a result of his fight for survival. He needed to have people touch him and be near him. It also gave him more control of his activities, such as being able to walk around the unit and walk to the room down the hall to see Scott Dudley. These things may seem insignificant, but when one's environment becomes that small these factors become very large in proportion.

JUNE 27, 1992—SATURDAY

(MEDICAL RECORDS) <u>Patient dozing at interval. Up riding stationary bicycle. Strong impression of a young person fighting sleep. Receiving morphine for pain. Mouth red and swollen with minimal bleeding. Lips red and swollen. Nausea and diarrhea. Temperature 100.5 F. Blood cultures drawn.</u>

(IVA) The problem now is mouth soreness — "dry and hurting." Mucositis is increasing. He is rinsing about every half hour with saline, also found out that rinsing with Sprite "feels good." Jack had two units of blood and platelets. He showered and walked around the units several times today. Slept intermittently today. Using oxygen less.

As a nurse on an oncology unit, I thought I had seen mucositis, but I was not prepared for the severity that Jack would have to endure. The problem with the soreness and pain in his mouth became the central focus of his day. He was constantly doing mouth care. When Jack walked around the unit, it was not a casual walk but a struggle. His feet and legs were swollen and he could not walk without someone to lean on. It was not a leisurely walk, but another way for Jack to cope, and each step became a fight for his recovery.

(JACK'S REFLECTIONS) *On this day, we were again visited by our former neighbors, Cleda and Tom Galiotto. Tom and Iva were sitting near the bottom of my bed and Cleda was sitting beside me. After years of verbal sparing between Cleda and myself, I think she was surprised when I asked her if I could hold her hand. I simply needed to feel the touch of another person. Later that year I wrote in their Christmas card, "I must have really been sick to have wanted to hold Cleda's hand."*

JUNE 28, 1992—SUNDAY

(MEDICAL RECORDS) <u>Morphine PCA for mouth pain. Generalized peripheral edema. Still using oxygen intermittently.</u>

(IVA) Jack called this morning, first time since he has been in the hospital. Feels better, mouth still sore. He showered this morning after having his head shaved by the nurse. He walked around the unit two times. Chris is here; he is real good with Jack. Jack received platelets and two units of blood (for anemia) today. Napping between longer intervals of being awake. Ate cream of wheat for breakfast. First food in about eight days. We took two more laps around the unit in the afternoon.

When Jack's hair began to fall out from the chemotherapy, his nurse suggested that he have his head shaved to eliminate the problem of having his hair all over his bed and clothing.

(JACK'S RECOLLECTIONS) *It is appropriate to give a description of my room at the Hutch. On the outside of the door to my room was a poster my daughter Karen had made. It had balloons and stars around a label indicating that the "Jackster" was inside. Beside the entrance to my door, was a place to insert photographs, where Iva had placed pictures of our family at Scott and Danielle's wedding. On the wall across from my bed, my daughter had placed a collage of photographs of our family and friends. If I ever had any doubts about the joys of life, they were quickly dispelled by a glance at that wall. The remaining walls of my room were covered with the cards we had received. I would not let anyone close the curtains, for I wanted my room to be bright and always tried to keep music playing. One of my nurses told me that when you entered my room there was an atmosphere of living and life.*

Prior to leaving for Seattle, I had recorded a collection of tapes of my favorite songs. In addition, many friends had also made tapes for me. Chris, my son, made a tape which included "What a Wonderful World" by Louis Armstrong. It was my favorite. Each time I heard it, I would remember sitting in Chris' room at home, sharing our thoughts as he was preparing the tape for me.

JUNE 29, 1992—MONDAY

(MEDICAL RECORDS) Patient is irritable. Realizes pain level will get worse before it gets better. Placed on fluid restriction. Temperature 101.4 F with chills. Blood cultures drawn.

(IVA) Rained last night. Still raining this morning and cooler. Jack slept through the night getting
up just to go to bathroom when needed. Mucositis
increasing. Jack does have VOD. Weight is also up
and there is some swelling in feet and ankles. Jack
walked two times around the unit this morning, showered, and went back to bed. I came back to the apartment about 2:30 PM to do laundry. Jack has a fever.
Blood cultures were drawn. Ate dinner at Swedish
Hospital with Jack's parents and Chris. Then went to
visit Jack at 6:30 PM. He walked around the unit
two more times. Chris and I talked to Jack's physician who told us he still has fluid in his lungs. Chris
and I came home at 9:00 PM and watched the video
he made here. He leaves tomorrow with Jack's parents.

Part of our daily routine was for me to assist Jack in the
morning with his shower. His nurse would place a chair and
the necessary towels in the shower which was located down
the hall from his room. Depending on his strength, he would
wash himself, or I would help him if he needed my assistance. I tried to do only as much as he wanted me to do. I
knew he needed and wanted to be able to do these tasks for
himself. After he showered, he would pause and rest before
drying himself. He then would rest again before putting on a
clean set of scrub clothes, which was followed by another
rest period before walking back to his room. When we returned to his room, I would put lotion and creams on his arms
and legs to prevent cracking of the skin and sores.

(JACK's RECOLLECTIONS) *When I could no longer
wear my tennis shoes (even with the laces removed), Iva arranged for me to get a pair of orthopedic boots, the kind worn*

on your feet over casts. Amazingly, they just fit my swollen feet. I used these boots to continue my daily walks. I believed that if I lay in bed, my body would be more susceptible to various infections and pneumonia. On most of my walks around the unit I would have one of my children on one side and Iva on the other side for support. One of the phenomena I experienced was a gradual shrinking of my world when I stayed in my room. This scared me because it was so easy to lie in my bed and watch the world gradually disappear. My walks enabled me to see other sections of the floor, other patients, and most importantly, other views of the outside world.

JUNE 30, 1992—TUESDAY

(MEDICAL RECORDS) Started continuous morphine infusion in addition to morphine PCA. Continued fluid restriction, Mouth and tongue painful, bleeding from lips and roof of mouth. Patient temperature 102.0 F after using ice packs. Throat cultures taken, Intermittent use of oxygen. Emesis dark brown and bloody.

> (IVA) Jack's parents and Chris left today and Karen arrived. She gave platelets and Jack received them. Today is day six post BMT.

Ice packs were placed between Jack's legs, under each arm, and at the back of his neck. These were used to help bring down his fever.

(JACK'S RECOLLECTIONS) *A person at this stage*

80

post-transplant is not a pretty site. The steroids and the lack of exercise stripped away my muscles. I had lost my hair and my skin had a red tone. I would eventually lose my finger-nails and toenails and my skin would peel off in long strips. My weight ballooned from 182 to 212 pounds, due to the retention of fluid. I looked into the mirror one day, and seeing my swollen lips and stomach, bald head, and stick-like arms and legs, I said to Iva that I looked just like the Grinch that stole Christmas.

When my son Chris first visited me on his second trip to Seattle, Iva found him slumped on the floor outside my room. He said he had become faint after seeing me, and said he never thought I would look that bad. I think in many ways my transplant was harder on my family then it was on me.

JULY 1, 1992—WEDNESDAY

(MEDICAL RECORDS) <u>Patient temperature 102.2 F Tongue oozing blood. Can't lay flat on bed due to mucus buildup and difficulty breathing. Lips swollen and bleeding. Nausea and vomiting.</u>

    (IVA) Mucositis continues. Elevated temperature.

When Jack was not doing well, the entries in my journal were limited. It was very difficult for me to accept what was happening to him and, if I wrote what was transpiring I was acknowledging these events. I therefore often chose, even in my telephone conversations with people at home, not to state his true condition.

(JACK'S RECOLLECTINS) *I seemed to be cold all of the time. I loved the blankets brought to me from the blanket warmer. Often I experienced violent shaking from being cold. Once I remember sitting on the bed with warm blankets on me, with Iva hugging me on one side and Karen hugging me on the other. All three of us were vibrating as I continued to shake. Today we laugh about that episode.*

JULY 2, 1992—THURSDAY

(MEDICAL RECORDS) <u>Patient has elevated kidney functions. Temperature 102.2 F. Blood cultures drawn. Cooling blanket placed on patient. Mouth is red and swollen.</u>

(IVA) Karen donated platelets. Elevated temperature.

As Jack continued to have a fever and chills, I became concerned that he would not get better. Those days and nights blended together. It seemed like an eternity.

(JACK'S RECOLLECTIONS) *I am not sure of the day (during this time I had very few lucid minutes), but I do remember waking up one night and seeing Iva and Karen sleeping in a chair wearing their surgical masks. I cried as I realized what my family was going through.*

JULY 3, 1992—FRIDAY

(MEDICAL RECORDS) <u>Patient edema increasing. Temperature 102.2 F. Weight increasing, retaining fluid. Kidney functions continue to be elevated. Renal consult ordered. Patient received two units of blood. Lips and face swollen. Increasing use of morphine PCA. Respiration rate increasing. Sputum cultures taken. Tissue breaking down on elbows.</u>

> **(IVA)** Karen donated platelets again. Jack is sleeping a lot during the day. Mucositis is really bad. Karen saying good-bye to Jack was very emotional. She will leave tomorrow.

Jack's appearance changed so dramatically that he hardly ever looked like himself. At this point, due to his mouth soreness, he was unable to speak. I became his voice and would answer the questions asked of him by the nurses and doctors. I think he got a little frustrated with me because, even after he could talk again, I continued to answer for him.

"Patient controlled anesthesia (PCA) the patient administers their own pain medications within the limits set by the nurse on the special pump."

<u>**Patient reference manual, Fred Hutchinson Cancer Research Center.**</u>

(JACK'S RECOLLECTIONS) *On my return visit to Seattle for a one-year recheck, one of my nurses commented that mine was the second worst case of mucositis that she had seen in her five years at the Hutch. Due to the deterioration of my skin tissue, I also developed open sores the size of a* *quarter on my elbows. These were treated with a bandage in the shape of a sleeve that was placed over my arms.*

JULY 4, 1992—SATURDAY

(MEDICAL RECORDS) Patient fever continues with chills. Feet are more swollen, weight increasing, edema worsening. Roof of mouth raw, swelling increasing in lips. Oral airway placed at bedside. Patient continues to suction mucus from mouth. Vigorous care of mouth by patient. Sputum cultures positive. Abdomen increasing in girth. Received one unit of red blood cells and platelets. Wife, realizing the serious condition of patient, is asking proper questions.

(IVA) A quiet 4th. Karen left early this morning. I went to the Hutch right after the airport. Stayed all day with Jack until 10:00 PM.

I began to accept the fact that Jack's life was in jeopardy, and I tried to get any type of reassurance from his nurse that I could. His nurse, knowing that I also was a nurse and that I was aware of the stress and strain that Jack's body was undergoing, could only say that his survival could go either way. As his condition continued to worsen, I kept thinking that his chances of survival were also decreasing. Jack's compulsion with his mouth care was unbelievable and became a topic of discussion with the nurses on the unit. It had to be seen to be believed.

(JACK'S RECOLLECTIONS) *I spent most of my wakening hours performing mouth care. I was either applying medications to my tongue, gargling medications for my mouth, or applying creams to my lips. When I wasn't doing these procedures, I was soaking my mouth and lips with ice water. The tray table beside my bed was covered with all of the medications and basins I needed for my mouth care. They were arranged in the order that I would use them. No one, not even Iva, was permitted to rearrange or tamper with the items on this tray table. When I was soaking my mouth and lips to lessen the pain and decrease the swelling, I had two basins on the tray. One was filled with crushed ice and the other one with cold water. I would mix the two together until I had just the right consistency of ice and water. I would then soak towels in this mixture and place them on my face and lips. I continued this procedure for hours.*

JULY 5, 1992—SUNDAY

(MEDICAL RECORDS) Patient temperature 102.4 F. Ice packs placed on patient. Plaque throughout mouth, tongue swollen. Patient mouth care continuing. Patient sitting in cardiac chair most of the day, trouble breathing when lying flat. Body red, petechia noted on abdomen and legs. Kidney functions remain elevated.

(IVA) Jack is having so much pain with his mouth. It is terrible to watch. Also elevated BUN, creatinine, and bilirubin. I am staying the night.

At this point, I was becoming even more concerned about Jack's deteriorating condition. He was not improving and I wasn't sure that he ever would. Once again, Jeanne was there

85

giving me the support and encouragement I needed.

(JACK'S RECOLLECTIONS) *I was on a morphine drip for the mouth pain. During this time I had visits from the pain control doctors. They would ask me a series of questions to determine whether I was receiving too much pain medication. Most often it was simple addition or subtraction of two digit numbers or they would tell me three words and then ask me to repeat those words at the end of the session. You can't imagine how challenging these simple tasks were. It was four or five months after the transplant before I was able to read a sentence. My mind had little ability to concentrate. For months after the transplant I would stare for prolonged periods of time. It was as if my mind would temporarily shut down. In many aspects, I had to retrain my mind to think in logical terms or normal problem solving methods. I remember the time a few months after we came home to Greensburg when the belt came off our self-propelled lawn mower. I was overwhelmed by the problem. The simple task of reattaching the belt took a great deal of analysis. I remember entering the house and telling Iva, excitedly, "I can fix things again."*

JULY 6, 1992—MONDAY

(MEDICAL RECORDS) Patient doing frequent, almost compulsive, mouthcare. Mouth swollen and raw, tongue raw on surface. Wife made observation, he seems to be afraid to sleep. Wiped tongue with tissue, large piece of tongue came off. Patient complains of mouth pain, but said, "it is under control." Temp 102.2 F.

(IVA) I went to the airport to meet my parents after spending the night with Jack. He had a very restless night, and I am tired. Mom and Dad arrived safely and enjoyed their plane ride.

I often was so tired I just wanted to crawl into bed, but the commitment to Jack and the family members who visited us, precluded my own needs. I guess each of us finds the reservoir of energy we need in these types of events in our lives.

(JACK's RECOLLECTIONS) *During this time my physician would place his hand on my abdomen, and with his fingers, measure from my rib, the extent of the swelling of my liver from the VOD. It all seemed like a dream to me.*

JULY 7, 1992—TUESDAY

(MEDICAL RECORDS) Patient oriented when questioned, increasingly anxious and a bit irritable. Tongue continues swollen and raw, has area 1/3" square with more bleeding. Platelets given. Blood in urine and stool. Feet purple from edema. Red raised rash over entire body

(IVA) Jack's renal and liver functions are not improving. He has so much mucositis and is not sleeping much at all. Also has GVHD (graft-versus-host disease) rash.

Throughout Jack's stay in Seattle, my role as a nurse and the support I gave him as his wife were often interchangeable. But an event on this day caused me to be unable to do either one. Jack's nurse and I were in his room when it was

87

apparent that he was having severe mouth pain. He tried to tell us what was happening, but we couldn't understand what he was saying. He then reached for a drinking cup from his tray and tried to scrape off a blood clot that was partially torn from his tongue. I knew he needed my help, but at this point I said, "I can't do this," and left the room. Using scissors, his nurse was able to cut the clot away from his tongue. At times, I found the conflict of being a nurse and wanting to care for him, and feeling the emotions and sadness as his wife, almost paralyzing.

JULY 8, 1992—WEDNESDAY

(MEDICAL RECORDS) <u>Tongue sloughing off at tip. Two pockets on tongue filled with dried blood. Platelets given. Femoral catheter bleeding, sandbag applied for pressure. Feet are grossly edematous. Patient admits to occasional confusion. Patient continues to sleep very little.</u>

(IVA) Jack started renal dialysis today due to kidney failure. Dialysis nurse was in and explained what they would be doing. The surgeon inserted a dialysis catheter in the right groin. I picked up Scott at 3:50 PM at the airport. We had our first polys today: 60!

This day was filled with mixed emotions. I was elated to learn that Jack's new bone marrow was producing cells, but at the same time, concerned that his organ failure was continuing and worsening.

"Polys - Another name for granulocytes or the white blood cells that fight bacterial infections."

88

Patient reference manual, Fred Hutchinson Cancer Research Center.

(JACK'S RECOLLECTIONS) *I received the news of the polys while sitting in a chair taking a shower. One of my favorite nurses burst in the door, pulled opened the shower curtain and said, "Guess what? You have polys," and got soaked while hugging me. This was the first indication that my son's bone marrow was producing new cells in my body (engraftment). Day 14 after the transplant.*

JULY 9, 1992—THURSDAY

(MEDICAL RECORDS) <u>Slight oozing from lower lip, stopped with pressure. Blood blister on tongue. Diarrhea. Given platelets in morning and afternoon. Bleeding at tip of tongue. Blood in urine and stool.</u>

(IVA) Scott donated platelets today. Dialysis was done from 7:30 AM to 10:30 AM. Cards, letters, and phone calls keep pouring in. People seem to know when we need it the most.

I knew that if Jack went into total kidney failure, he could only survive a few more days, I prayed that his kidney functions would reverse the gradual deterioration that had occurred over the last week. The cards and letters helped to keep my spirit up. I felt that we were really not so far from everyone, and each card expressed love and concern for us and told us that we were in their prayers.

JULY 10, 1992—FRIDAY

(MEDICAL RECORDS) Patient received platelets in morning and afternoon. Mouth, tongue and lips continue to bleed. Blood oozing from right side of nostril. Increasing thick mucus in mouth. Scabs developing on tongue. Underside of tongue very sore. Wife and son/donor present at bedside. Both are very supportive and helpful. Family very appropriate with expectations. Taking things as they are in the present. Wife and son alternating visits-making sure they get their rest.

(IVA) Jack had dialysis again today. He usually sleeps through the procedure. Platelets are only 2,000 with bleeding during the night from his tongue. Scott donated platelets again today. Jack has also received single donor platelets for the first time. I love you, Jack.

I began to prepare myself for the very real possibility that Jack may die. I thought about what I would say to our parents, and finally, what I would tell our children. I knew Jack wouldn't give up, but I hoped that if he wasn't going to survive that he wouldn't remain in this condition for a long period of time. That would be the last thing he would want.

JULY 11, 1992—SATURDAY

(MEDICAL RECORDS) Patient received two units of platelets. Rash improving, skin peeling. Kidney functions improving. Scabs increasing on tongue. No bleeding on tongue.

(IVA) They gave Scott the day off. (He didn't donate platelets) Jack's skin is starting to improve. Fingers peeling. Head and neck also peeling Mouth greatly improved. Scott, Mom, and Dad went to Pike Street Market and dinner. Jack had dialysis and more platelets.

On this day, the levels of Jack's kidney functions began to drop dramatically toward the normal range. I began thinking: He is going to do it; he really is going to make it back!

JULY 12, 1992—SUNDAY

(MEDICAL RECORDS) Glucose up, patient given insulin. Face ruddy, rash decreasing. Skin continues to peel off. Mouth improving. Patient walked around the unit, quickly fatigued.

(IVA) No dialysis today! Scott gave platelets for the fourth time. Jack went outside today for about twenty minutes. He is having some diarrhea. This evening Scott and I took Mom and Dad to the top of the Space Needle.

I was elated, but I was also emotionally and physically exhausted. I thought: If he can make it through this crisis with his kidneys, then he is strong enough to conquer whatever lies ahead of him.

(JACK'S RECOLLECTIONS) *For me, this was a monumental day. When my nurse told me I could go outside, I felt like a little child. I couldn't get ready fast enough. Bundled with warm towels around my head, blankets around my body,* *and a surgical mask on my face I was placed in a wheelchair and pushed outside by my father-in-law. To see the flowers, smell the air, and to feel the wind on my face was emotionally overwhelming. I will never forget that day! Those few minutes reaffirmed my desire to fight for my life. Whoever suggested this outing obviously had some insight into the positive effect it would have on me.*

JULY 13, 1992—MONDAY

(MEDICAL REPORTS) <u>Mouth improving, lips cracked and bleeding slightly. Kidney functions continue to improve.</u>

(IVA) Jack is starting to sleep better. I took Mom and Dad to the airport. Jack had platelets again. He is continuing to improve. Received flowers from the girls I work with at home. I miss them. We watched the video that Chris put together of our slides from England. Amazing how the kids have grown. Talked by phone to Karen and Chris at home. Everyone sounds well. Jack tried tapioca pudding and it stayed down!

(JACK'S RECOLLECTIONS) *One of the few items that I had been able to eat was something the employees of the Hutch called a "slushy." I guess it was frozen Kool-Aid in a small plastic cup. Whenever one was delivered to my room, which was three or four times a day, I would stir it to the right consistency as it thawed. Later, my family said I almost drove them crazy with my compulsive stirring. This evening I asked for my favorite orange "slushy" and was told they had none in the kitchen. I asked for my second flavor choice and was told they were totally out of "slushies." I received the same story the following morning.*

92

Each morning an entourage of physicians and allied health professionals would visit me. The group of perhaps six to nine people would confer outside my room to discuss my case before entering. On this particular morning, as they held their hallway conference, I was preparing my "slushy" speech (as it was later called) for them. When I was asked how I was doing, I said, "Not well!" I realized this was a big institution with many priorities, but at this time, I had only one: to receive a "slushy" when I asked for it. I wanted someone to explain to me why I was having a problem. My little outburst prompted considerable laughter in the group. One of the physicians turned to my nurse and said, "I think he's better."

JULY 14, 1992—TUESDAY

(MEDICAL RECORDS) Patient blood pressure elevated, complains of being hungry. Glucose continues elevated, received insulin. Patient's mood reserved optimism. Flat affect about doing better. States he has been through too much to allow himself to become excited right now.

(IVA) Jack is staying about the same with his blood counts. Will receive community platelets this morning. Scott will give platelets in the afternoon for Jack. Edema in the ankles and feet is decreasing. Skin rash is fading. Jack went out on a pass to our apartment from 3:00 PM. to 6:00 PM. He exercised when we came back. He had a good day.

I watched him push himself to exercise in the physical therapy room, using the stationary bicycle and dumbbells. Jack's nurse kept saying to me that there is "no quit" in this guy.

(JACK'S RECOLLECTIONS) *On my floor at the Hutch was a small room devoted to physical therapy. It had a stationary bicycle, a treadmill and some small dumbbells. My physical*

93

therapist was great. I loved the room because I could look out the window and see oak trees, beds of ivy, and lots of flowers.

JULY 15, 1992—WEDNESDAY

(MEDICAL RECORDS) Patient getting more excited about going home. At 2040 patient seen seizing by wife. At 2043 multiple nurses in room, seizure subsided. Placed on Dilatin for seizures.

(IVA) Jack ate cream of wheat with milk for his breakfast. He was up at 7:30 AM and exercised on the treadmill. Walked two times around the unit before his morning shower. Jack will be going out on a pass again today. Everyone is amazed at how well he is doing. He walked two more times around the unit before going out on the pass to our apartment. Went to the apartment on the van and then we took a walk up to the corner of Broadway and Boren. Sat on a bench under a tree and looked at Mt. Rainier. When we returned to the apartment, Jack took a nap. He later ate tapioca pudding and drank grape soda. He tried macaroni and cheese, but couldn't eat it. Scott drove us back to the Hutch. He leaves tomorrow. Scott returned to the apartment to pack. I stayed with Jack and we walked one time around the unit. Jack went into his room and sat down on a chair and began having a seizure. Scott came back to the Hutch after I called him. Jack had a CT brain scan and stat labs. Seen by doctor on call. CT scan negative. Labs okay. I spent the night with him.

(JACK'S RECOLLECTIONS) *There are many days during my hospitalization of which I have no recollection of any events. But this day I remember vividly. I think it was one of the* *major turning points in my recovery. I can just imagine what a sight I was walking the streets of Seattle in my blue orthopedic boots, surgical mask, jacket and wool hat in the midst of summer. I was always so cold. Occasionally, after the transplant, my mind would begin to race. Every thought seemed to accelerate through my brain. Prior to this day I was able to slow down my thoughts and bring things back to normal speed. Following my walk around the unit, I felt my mind speeding and began to feel dizzy. Fortunately, I was near my room and I immediately went in and sat down in a chair. The next thing I was aware of was lying in bed receiving oxygen. I looked at Iva and she said I had a seizure. I told her I could hear her voice. She said that was impossible. I then repeated her words back to her. She had first pleaded with me not to die and to hang on. She then asked God to keep me alive. Even with more than half a dozen people in the room, many of them giving instructions on my care, I was still able to pick out her voice. If ever two people connected, it was "us" on that day. When Iva heard her words repeated, she began to cry, followed by tears from the nurses in the room. A very emotional time for everyone. A year later, when I returned to Seattle for a check-up, the nurses who were in the room that day recounted the events with continued amazement.*

JULY 16, 1992—THURSDAY

(MEDICAL RECORDS) Patient mouth clear, tongue healing, ridge of tongue still with redness and slight breakdown. No further seizures. Wife spent all night with patient; he was extremely frightened by the events of the previous night.

(IVA) Returned to the apartment at 5:30 AM and

took Scott to airport. Arrived at Hutch at 8:30 AM.
Jack doing okay. He slept most of the day; awake a few
minutes at a time to go to the bathroom or drink fluids.
Scott called from Pittsburgh on his way home to see if
Jack was okay. We walked around the unit this evening.

JULY 17, 1992—FRIDAY

(MEDICAL RECORDS) Patient more active. Mouth continues to improve. Kidney and liver functions improving.

> **(IVA)** Jack is much better today. There have been
> no further seizures. Jack rode stationary bike 0.9 miles.
> Walked around the unit eight times today. Physical
> therapy for exercising. More awake today. Bone mar-
> row biopsy results in today. Marrow 60% engraftment.
> Good news! Jack received platelets today.

The speed of Jack's recovery was described by one of his
nurses as a miracle. In a matter of days he went from one of the
sickest patients on the unit to a patient whose discharge from the
Hutch was being planned.

JULY 18, 1992—SATURDAY

(MEDICAL RECORDS) Patient able to drink. Tip of tongue
improving.

> **(IVA)** Jack is feeling better, rode his bike two miles
> today. Jack again was out on a pass; we spent four
> hours together at the apartment. He started on the

96

medicine cyclosporine today. His blood counts continue to improve.

JULY 19, 1992—SUNDAY

(MEDICAL RECORDS) <u>Patient up walking around unit at 0800. Patient out on pass, returned in good spirits.</u>

> **(IVA)** Out on pass most of the day. Returned in the afternoon for Jack to receive platelets. Took a drive down to Lake Union. Returned to the Hutch at 7:00 PM.

(JACK'S RECOLLECTIONS) *On this day I began to take down the cards and letters we had received and the collage of photographs that Karen had placed on the walls of my room. When my doctor entered my room and observed what I was doing, he commented that he guessed I was preparing to leave.*

JULY 20, 1992—MONDAY

(MEDICAL RECORDS) <u>Discharge planning and teaching discussed with patient and wife. Patient unable to sleep due to excitement.</u>

> **(IVA)** Jack is continuing to improve. Out on pass again—to be discharged tomorrow.

JULY 21, 1992—TUESDAY

(IVA) Discharged at 10:00 AM! We came back
to the apartment and both of us took a nap.

(JACK'S RECOLLECTIONS) *A couple weeks before I
left for Seattle, Iva and I bumped into an aquaintance at a
local restaurant. She had heard that I was going to Seattle
for a transplant. She told me to say hello to Him while I was
in the northwest.*

*"Him? I questioned. Who is he? Do you know someone in
Seattle?"*

*She said, "I'm talking about God; I'm sure that you'll be
talking to Him a lot."*

*She was correct, I prayed for my recovery, but most of all I
prayed for my family who was suffering with me.*

CHAPTER VI

My Journey

I believe there were four factors that helped me survive the transplant. First there was the will of God and the combination of the prayers said on my behalf. Then there was Iva's touch. There were many days when this was the only sensory stimulation I received. I could not hear or see anything, but I could feel her holding my hand. At night she would sleep bent over in a chair, with her head on my bed. My hand would occasionally touch her head as she slept. That touch was crucial to me; it was my contact and link with the world. I kept thinking, *That's Iva and she's still here.*

A third factor was my determination to exercise whenever possible. I strived to increase my strength by increasing the number of times I could walk around the unit and the amount of miles I could ride on my stationary bicycle. As each increased, I felt a sense of accomplishment and progress. I was getting stronger!

The final and a very important vehicle for my recovery was what I was able to do in my mind, through what I refer to as "my journey." I believe my journey began July 9, 1992 and ended July 11, 1992. This was the time of my hospitalization when my condition was the most critical.

Even with the pain medications I was receiving, my mind

was able to review my life and the joys of living. Prior to leaving for Seattle, I had thought about this mental journey; however, at no time did I think that this activity would be so instrumental in my survival and recovery. The vivid recollection of past places and people in my life was drawn from memories I thought I had long forgotten.

The journey I took was a mental walk through my life. On this walk, darkness and death lay behind me. Ahead were light and life. At times I felt the sensation of slipping back into a crevice of darkness. I had to keep walking toward the light and my life in order to stay alive. A week before we left Seattle to return home, one of my physicians said to me, "You came as close to the edge as you can come." I found the symbolism of his statement remarkably similar with what I call the "dark times" of my recovery.

My first "stop" on my mental journey back to life was the Episcopal church in my hometown of Follansbee, West Virginia. In my mind I was walking down the aisle of the church, carrying the cross in the Christmas service processional. Our church was very small and, in my vision, the processional consisted of only the Vicar and me. He was the first of many people who would join me on my journey back. When we arrived at the altar, I lit the candles on each side and, because it was Christmas, I also lit the communion candle.

In "real" life, I had served as the church's only crucifer and acolyte for four years. In my life, the Vicar probably had the greatest influence on who I am today. From my bed at the Hutch, I thought about the talks we had in his office before the services. He shared his philosophy of life and happiness. Over his lifetime he was a millionaire and an alcoholic, eventually becoming penniless, before he turned to the priesthood. As an Episcopal priest he gave his salary to people who he felt needed it more than he did. Often he would eat at our house when he couldn't afford to buy food. His perception of life was to always look for the good in people and situations.

He taught me the joys of giving and the rewards of caring for people. He also taught me that, no matter what the hardship, each of us has the ability to succeed. He had very few material possessions, but he viewed his life as a success and he was happy.

Each Christmas the Vicar would give the same sermon about the little girl whose father was an alcoholic. Her Christmas wish was that her father would stop "smelling of prunes." I relived that sermon in my mental journey. Then, during communion, I felt his hand as he placed it on my forehead and made the sign of the cross. His hands were like none I had ever experienced before. This was a man who carried a sense of warmth in his touch.

Throughout my spiritual and mental journey, the hands of people who joined me in my vision were in concert with the touch of Iva as she clutched my hand in Room 74 of the Fred Hutchinson Cancer Research Center. Her hands were my anchor to life.

During the church service, I would kneel at the altar on a wooden step. During particularly long services, like Christmas, it would become very uncomfortable. When I would complain, Vicar would say, "Just think how much character you are building." I often used that same phrase with my children when they were doing a positive task that was exceedingly unpleasant. Finally, I thought about the only personal item that I had packed for my trip to Seattle: a Book of Common Prayer given to me by the Vicar. The inscription dated February 16, 1956 read, "To Jack—The good and faithful cross bearer. I am your true friend." It was signed, "Theodore Hubbell." This man was much more than a friend; he was a mentor and inspiration for a nine-year-old boy. The memory of the greatness of this humble man carried me to the next stop of my mental journey.

In my mind, I was walking through a cornfield to the pond at my Aunt Rose and Uncle Bud's farm in Chairton, Iowa.

Although they were actually my great aunt and uncle, it seemed natural for me to refer to them as my aunt and uncle. As I passed through the field with my bamboo fishing pole over my shoulder, carrying a can of worms, and constantly watching not to step on a bull snake, I could hear the wind whistling through the corn stalks. The wind seemed to blow continually in Iowa. With only the worms, bamboo pole, line and hook, you could catch sunfish all day at the pond. As I neared the pond I could see the heads of the snapping turtles on the surface of the water. In the "old days" when we caught one of these snappers, Dad would make delicious turtle soup. My mental image of the sun shining on me while I was sitting in the grass with my line in the water, diligently watching the float, was as close to being there as possible. What a tranquil place for a young boy to lull away the hours! In my vision, I could see the figures of Mom and Aunt Rose in the kitchen while I was walking back to the farm house. As I entered the back porch I could hear the sizzling sounds, and smell the wonderful aroma of chicken frying.

In my journey, when we sat down to dinner, Aunt Rose was to my right where she always sat in order to make sure that I ate all my food. I was always a thin child and Aunt Rose had taken on the task of fattening me up. Uncle Bud was at the head of the table talking about Aunt Rose's "stack" gravy, so-called because everyone said it could stand on its own. My vision of this scene from the late 1950's was extremely vivid. I was even hiding the peas under my plate, as I so often did thirty-five years earlier. (I still don't like peas.)

After dinner we relaxed in the living room as Uncle Bud pulled out his pocket watch, lit up his pipe, and checked if the Rock Island railroad train was on schedule as it passed the house. As my mind traveled back to this time, I remember thinking frequently as a young boy, *What an awfully boring place this is.* In my vision, however, it was a place of tranquillity and peace as I lay on the floor, watching Uncle

Bud sit in his rocking chair, smoking his pipe. That same oak rocking chair now sits in our bedroom.

When I began to recover, one of the first things I asked Iva to do was to find out where everyone actually sat at Uncle Bud's house during dinner. When I asked her to call my mom and dad for the seating arrangements, I think she thought I had probably lost my marbles. This was a time when I was prone to staring into space for long periods of time. When Iva reported the results of her inquiry, I was elated to know that my vision of the dinner table during my journey was exactly as it had been thirty-five years before!

Many years later, when the farm was being sold at auction after Uncle Bud and Aunt Rose passed away, I knelt in the farm house bedroom where I had slept as a young boy and thanked them for my wonderful memories. I couldn't imagine a more pleasurable place for a young boy to spend his summers. I ended my mental journey to Iowa, holding hands with Aunt Rose as we walked around the courthouse square in town. As a young teenager, I was always embarrassed when she held my hand when we went shopping. Now, I welcomed her touch and the recollection of it in my life.

My next stop on my journey was the backyard of my childhood home. Each summer as a youth I would eagerly await the arrival of Uncle Don and Aunt Mary, and my cousins Donna and Mark, from California. Their arrival always prompted a cookout at our house. As I looked around the yard in my mental journey, Dad was cooking hamburgers on the sheet of stainless steel that he had placed over the brick fireplace. He was adding his special seasoning of hot peppers and tomatoes. Beside the house, Mark and my other cousins, Lee and Larry, were playing badminton with Uncle Don. My sister Jeanne and my cousin Donna were sitting on the swing under the vine-covered trellis. My Uncle Les was harassing Dad about his seasoning. Grandma, Aunt Harriet, Aunt Mary, and my mother were trying to set the table. My mother always seemed to be a little bit unorganized, but as I looked back now, that was part of her relaxed personality that everyone loved. My brother Jim and I were playing wiffle ball in front of the garage.

After eating, Mom and I were sitting next to each other at the picnic table doing our old hand slapping routine: She would place her hand above mine and I would slap her hand upward. (I have seen movies of Mom and I doing this same thing when I was only two or three years old.) That image of a silly gesture of my mother and me playing with each others hands moved me to the next stop on my journey.

Now seventeen, I was walking up a tree-lined street in Wellsburg, West Virginia, with my first "girlfriend." Carol and I were walking from her house to the Dairy Queen. As we walked back eating ice cream cones, holding hands, and enjoying the Ohio Valley summer, the memory of that innocent time, brought me a great feeling of happiness. On Sunday afternoons when her parents were visiting relatives, we were not permitted in the house. On those days, we would spend the afternoon sitting on the glider on her front porch while the rest of the concerned residents on the street watched us.

The first adult experience on my mental journey was a visit to my fraternity house in college. With me were my three friends, all named Dave: Dave #1 (nicknamed, Alka), Dave #2 (nicknamed, Thuts) and then "just plain" Dave. We were a group of young men who displayed the joys of youth and clean honest fun. As we shared college life, we genuinely enjoyed each other's support and friendship. I am sure that as I lay in my bed in the Hutch unaware of my surroundings, reliving this experience, there must have been a smile on my face. Although Thuts and Alka were large men, they both had a sense of gentleness and kindness that made our friendship special. A month before the transplant I had sat down with these same three gentleman for dinner. They now had become a high school principal, a town mayor, and a director of human resources, respectively, all successful in their lives. As we shared the evening, I realized that the same joy for life and kindness that I found so attractive in these men as college friends was still evident in their lives. We vowed to return to that same restaurant when I returned from Seattle.

The next journey was to the Outer Banks of North Carolina. With great joy and peace, I was sitting on the beach with Iva, watching our children playing in the ocean. They were young at this recollection, Scott had not yet entered his teens. I could see the pelicans flying by in a row, skimming the top of the water, as sea birds ran back and forth dodging the surf. Now, in the water, Scott and I lay on our surf riders waiting for a good wave. With pride and enormous love, I watched Iva, Karen, and Chris.

There were many other stops on my journey, involving a person or persons of great importance in my life. Each held vivid excitement and an appreciation for life. One short stop took me to the Border country of Scotland. I revisited the place that Scott and I had hiked to four years before. This was also a place of peace and supreme beauty. In my journey, we were walking through a glen near the top of Grey Mare's Tail, the highest waterfall in Scotland. With sheep grazing around me, I lay down looking up at the sun with tufts of sheep wool glistening in the heather around me. I repeated the statement that I had made four years earlier: "If there is a heaven, I want it to be just like this."

As if my mind knew that my body was recovering, the last place I visited was the backyard of our home in Greensburg, Pennsylvania. *I had returned to the present.* In my journey, Iva and I were walking towards the pool as the kids were swimming. As I stood there holding Iva's hand, the murmuring in my room became audible voices. The figures that were shadows became recognizable individuals.

My mental journey was over, it was July 11, 1992. My

spirit had walked my mind and body back to room 74 at the Fred Hutchinson Cancer Research Center in Seattle, Washington. Immediately, my condition began to improve and my nurses started to refer to me as the "miracle man." Now began my physical journey back.

I have heard many theories concerning the reason for my journey and the affect it had on my deteriorating physical condition. My pastor suggested that the walk through the events of my life was the recovery path that God laid out for me. He said His light had shown the direction and way for me. Others told me that my journey was a way of reaffirming my fight for my life by mentally reliving pleasurable episodes. Another theory is that, as my mind was enjoying all of these past activities, it caused my body to generate the same hormones that it did when I actually experienced these events. According to this theory, this rush of physically simulating hormones within my body activated the healing process that started my recovery.

Personally, I believe that the affects were brought about by a combination of all three theories.

CHAPTER VII

Summer in Seattle

Post-transplant

At this point, I have difficulty describing many of the emotions that accompanied my experiences in Seattle. Because of the extensive amount of medications I was receiving, my feelings and emotions were blunted, but the day that I was discharged from the Hutch was a day of exhilaration. Walking to the front door of the Hutch and passing through to the outside were moments filled with excitement. Walking over to the car, opening the door, and getting in brought tears to my eyes. *I truly was back in the outside world again.* This was not a pass. I was going back to our Seattle apartment to stay, and then, later, after my outpatient care was completed, I would be going home to Greensburg.

Leaving the Hutch was more than a simple matter of moving my care to a new setting. It was also an opportunity for me to again see Mt. Rainier in the horizon and to ride down to Elliott Bay and Lake Union. Of course each day included a trip to the Hutch outpatient center at 600 Broadway.

A typical day following my discharge began with Iva and me riding the van up to the outpatient facility, usually before

9:00 AM, where I would have blood drawn from my Hickman line for testing. Initially, we would ride the van back to the apartment; however, as I grew stronger, we would walk the four blocks back to First Hill Apartments. Although, at times, it was a nuisance to visit the outpatient facility every day, being so closely monitored brought great comfort and a sense of reassurance. We knew help was only minutes away.

In the afternoon we usually reported back to the outpatient facility where I would receive medication or, sometimes, blood products. The Hickman line in my chest was and would be my source of nutrition and hydration for the next few months. In the beginning, I was receiving some type of fluid through the line eighteen hours a day. The fluids (medication, nutrition, and hydration) were delivered through the catheter into my blood stream by the Provider pump. The pump was a small unit that, with its carrying case, probably weighed only a couple of pounds and measured approximately 10"x12." The carrying case also held the IV bag. So for most of the day the pump was my companion. Whenever I went for a walk, I would place the strap over my shoulder and run the line down through the top of my shirt. I soon learned that running suits with zipper fronts were the most practical outfits to wear.

Iva and I worked on different systems to enable me to take a shower or to sleep without being connected to the pump. It always seemed that I ended up going to bed with the line of the pump attached to my chest, and the Provider pump resting against the side of my bed.

Because of the amount of fluid I was receiving, I made frequent trips to the bathroom each night. Carrying my trusty pump with the line dangling down, I would set off for the bathroom. I tried not to turn on any light for fear of waking Iva. If I caught the line on something, I could feel it tugging at the entrance to my chest, an unusual sensation to say the least. I found that the best way to accomplish what I needed to do in the bathroom was to hang the Provider pump on the bathroom door knob.

When the pump had air in the line, or the IV bag was empty, an alarm would go off in the pump. This always seemed to occur in the middle of the night. As I lay in bed, Iva would flush the lines with a syringe to try to get the air out. Or, she would change the IV bag. It was months before Iva had the luxury of sleeping through the night. Even now, I sometimes hear the beeping sound of the pump when I'm dreaming.

My mouth continued to be a problem after I was discharged from the Hutch. The graft-versus-host disease and the mucositis had improved, but were still present. Eating became an event accompained by considerable discomfort. I started with soups, gelatins and puddings. Even these items caused severe pain. I would place a spoonful in my mouth and then grasp onto both arms of my chair as I swallowed. The joy of eating was lost in pain. Because my mouth was not improving, I was placed on a steroid mouthwash that I used daily to stimulate healing. I would stand in front of the sink in our apartment and place the prescribed dose in my mouth. Often I would end up on my knees, my face red and sweating, as I spit the liquid back into the sink. The pain was excruciating.

Although we were in Seattle, we were in daily contact with our family and friends at home. There was not a day during our stay that we did not receive a letter, card, or a telephone call with words of encouragement and support. These letters often included checks or cash.

Because I had been dealing with leukemia for such a long time, we had time to save and prepare for the expense of a transplant in a distant city. We were not in need of additional financial support. There were many others at the Hutch, however, who were not as blessed. Therefore, some of the funds we received from family and friends were given to other transplant families.

One of the most unusual items we received from home

was a poster prepared by Don Turnbull, a member of our church. It was great! The poster contained the photographs of our pastor, of Don, and six other members of our church. Below each photograph were written words of encouragement from the individual shown. But what made this poster truly unique was the fact that we received it in twenty-eight pieces. (Don had prepared the poster and then cut it into twenty-eight puzzle-shaped pieces). Because Don travels a great deal in his work, we received one piece every few days, mailed from various locations across the eastern United States. As we did, I would eagerly add each new piece to the puzzle. What a marvelous idea!

After my discharge from the Hutch, Iva would frequently express her desire to return to our home. Her phrase, "I want to go home" was heard by many of our friends in Pennsylvania. One of my former coworkers from Latrobe Hospital sent her a very small pair of ruby colored slippers. They were accompanied by a note stating that a similiar pair got a little girl back to Kansas and maybe this pair of slippers would help Iva get back to Pennsylvania.

Following my discharge from the Hutch, I was re-admitted twice to Swedish Hospital due to complications, each time for about a week. Once, in August, was for blood infections and the second time, in September, was for a blood clot in my right leg. Throughout my stay in Seattle, Iva's face was my barometer of how serious my condition was. When I was rushed to the hospital in August with four different types of blood infections, I immediately began having severe shakes and chills. Even with continued injections of demerol and warm blankets, my shaking would not stop. I remember looking at Iva's face and thinking that this was a time to worry.

I was discharged from the Hutch ten days before Scott Dudley. Initially, he and I spent most of our time in our apartments following our discharge. Jeanne and Iva would go on frequent trips to the grocery store and on periodic shopping expeditions. Scott and I tried to pursuade them to go out more and more and, when they did, they would place the two of us in the same room, with the idea that if one of us got into trouble the other could call the Hutch for help.

When Scott and I were strong enough, we resumed our sight-seeing tour of the Northwest, this time with masks covering our faces. On two occassions we journeyed to Snoqualmie Falls (now with either Jeanne or Iva driving) to enjoy the scenery. But my favorite excursion was down to the Pike Street Market to shop for fruit and to simply enjoy the atmosphere of this special place. I particularly enjoyed walking by the booths of cut flowers at the market. Iva kept fresh flowers in our apartment as often as possible because she realized how much I missed our gardens at home.

The Hutch had a policy that requested that the patient stay in the Seattle area for one hundred days, post-transplant. Prior to the transplant, that time seemed exceptionally long to me. Now, in view of the complications I experienced, I realize how dangerous it would have been for me to return home any earlier. It was also during that period that I had the opportunity to spend a great deal of time with other patients who had received bone marrow transplants. Each day we would meet at the treatment room at the outpatient facility. The treatment room was a large area filled with reclining chairs where we would spend hours receiving IV medications through our Hickman lines. It was also the place where we shared our dreams, hopes, and fears. Scott Dudley and I seemed to be on different medication schedules, so we were very seldom at the clinic at the same time. The people I most clearly remember were Becky, who wanted to get married and have children, Chloe, who wanted to be around for her grandchildren, and David, who told everyone that he simply wanted to get old like Jack. David, who challenged me emotionally, was nineteen years old with a row of studs along the length of one of his ears. At first, he was an intimidating figure for someone of my generation. Over time, however, we became friends, and would search for each other at the clinic so that we could sit in adjoining chairs. David's life was not one filled with a great deal of happiness. He had spent most of his life in various foster homes. I committed myself to helping him following my return home.

I looked for David when I returned to the outpatient facility following my second hospitalization at Swedish Hospital. When he wasn't there, I assumed I had missed him that day. On the second day when he didn't show up, I asked one of the nurses when David was scheduled to come in. Her response was that I should talk to one of the doctors. By this time I was getting anxious and started pressing for an answer. I was eventually told that David had died from a fungus infection while I was in the hospital. That day was very difficult for me. Becky died less than a week after returning to her home, and Chloe died while still in Seattle. I often think of my conversations in the treatment room and say a prayer for those who didn't survive and for the families they left behind. I continue to be troubled by the question of why some people made it and some didn't. Often there was no correlation between the extent of the patient's complications and his or her survival.

On September 23, 1992, four months after we arrived in Seattle, Iva and I went to the "Hutch" to say good-bye to the staff. After thanking everyone for providing me with such special care, I left Iva and walked around the unit by myself. This was a walk I had taken so many times in the past, often with a great deal of assistance from my family. With each step, my emotions continued to rise. When I, once again, reached the entrance to the unit and rejoined Iva, I looked up and said, "We did it!" I had a feeling of triumph that I will probably never duplicate in my life. We flew home to Pittsburgh the next day.

CHAPTER VIII

The Children's View

SCOTT

L ate in the summer of 1983, when I was fourteen years old, my father was diagnosed with leukemia. I wasn't sure then what leukemia was, just that my parents said Dad had a problem with creating too many bad white blood cells. I remember not knowing how or what to feel.

I was in eighth grade that fall. One day, as I sat in science class, a friend turned to me and said, "Sorry about your dad being sick." He went on to explain that he had heard from his mother that my father had leukemia and that people with leukemia didn't live very long. I was really confused. I didn't know what to say to him other than, "Thanks." Dad didn't really seem sick, except for being a little tired and worn down. And he certainly didn't act like someone who was going to die soon. It was hard for me to accept that he had leukemia and that people with leukemia only live for a limited amount of time. Dad never turned into a sickly invalid who required constant care, so, I guess, like the rest of my family, I just tried to put his illness out of my mind and went on with life.

My parents raised me with a lot of love and had given all their children everything they could. They met in college and were married young; my mother was nineteen and my father was twenty-two. A little over a year after their wedding in September 1969, I was born. Like many couples in the early stages of marriage, they didn't have much; therefore, any monetary gains were usually offset by supplying basic needs for the family. My sister, Karen, was born in October 1972, and my brother, Chris, in February 1975. The pressures of raising a family and the constant sacrifices entailed can place a great deal of strain on the relationship of any couple. As a result, during the late seventies and early eighties, my parents went through some very turbulent times. But, when my father was diagnosed with leukemia, it seemed to wipe the slate clean for them. I think knowing that my father could die in the near future made them realize just how important they were to each other. I don't know whether God allowed my father to have leukemia or, if He used it as a way of strengthening my parent's marriage; however, deep down inside, I believe that His intervention played a part in my father's illness and recovery.

Throughout my high school and college years, my father's health remained moderately good. He would occasionally need to take chemotherapy to lower his white blood cell count, but he maintained his normal life style and looked healthy. Inwardly, he must have felt a constant peril looming in the darkness. As a result, he was constantly planning how the family would be taken care of after he died. Although a gloomy thought, I think it gave him a great deal of satisfaction to know his family would be okay in his absence.

In 1991, I became engaged to my future wife, Danielle, and we started planning our wedding for the spring of the following year. During this period, my father's condition was continually worsening. When the chemotherapy began to lose its effectiveness, he started receiving interferon injections.

The interferon often brought on fevers and made Dad quite sick. Although there were some beneficial effects, his condition was still moving in the wrong direction. The doctors were pushing him to plan for a bone marrow transplant. It became clear that if he did not have one, he was going to die —not someday—but very soon.

Dad researched which hospitals were doing bone marrow transplants with patients who had his particular type of leukemia. The hospital with the best success rate was the Fred Hutchinson Cancer Center in Seattle, Washington. He and my mother traveled to Seattle for a consult in January 1992. They were told that they needed to get the ball rolling toward finding a donor and setting a tentative date for the transplant.

The doctors in Seattle wanted to test Dad's brother and sister, and his children. I was really hoping I could be the donor, although I wasn't keen about undergoing the procedure. My blood was drawn in Blacksburg, Virginia and sent to Seattle. Dad called me a few days later to give me the test results. His voice sounded strained, "Karen and you could be donors, although neither of you is a perfect match. You both have a five-out-of-six antigen match with me."

I was really excited and happy that they had found a possible donor and that it might be me. Even though Dad was grateful, he sounded concerned. He probably had reservations about one of his children donating the marrow, knowing that there would be physical discomfort and emotional stress. I had expected him to be happier.

In late January of 1992, my Dad was trying to set a date for the transplant. My wedding was scheduled for May 16, 1992. He really wanted to be at the wedding, but the doctors in Seattle were pushing him to schedule the procedure as soon as possible. If he scheduled the transplant in early spring, he would surely miss the wedding. The choice of having a life-saving procedure or attending a son's wedding might seem obvious to most people. I told him that it would be better if he missed the event and lived to see his grandchildren, rather than postpone the transplant and risk his life for the sake of attending my wedding. But Dad felt there was a chance he was going to die in Seattle and he wanted to see his son get married. For my parents and myself, planning the transplant and looking forward to my wedding at the same time brought happiness and sadness in constant flux.

We were scheduled to fly to Seattle two days after Danielle and I returned from our honeymoon. Our wedding day came and it was a glorious family celebration. The whole occasion was very upbeat and everybody had a good time. I tried to put out of my mind what lay ahead for my father.

When Danielle and I returned from the Cayman Islands following our honeymoon, I flew to Pittsburgh and met Mom and Dad for the flight to Seattle. Danielle was not able to come with us at that time because of her job (like my mother, she's a nurse). She had used up all of her vacation time for the wedding and our honeymoon.

My parents had rented an apartment in Seattle close to the Hutch. A lot of transplant patients and their families were also living in the building. The building was only a few blocks from the hospital. My dad's transplant date was postponed numerous times during our first week in Seattle. Dad, Mom, and I decided that I should fly home to Danielle until a definite date was set for his admittance to the hospital.

It was great to be back in Blacksburg with Danielle. She was so supportive of me and my family throughout the entire experience. We were apart more than we were together during the first few months of our marriage. Also, Dr. Simmons, who was mentoring my graduate program, gave me great latitude in my academic work which enabled me do what was necessary for my family. I will always be grateful for his support and understanding. I flew back to Seattle three days before Dad was to be admitted to the Hutch. Danielle soon followed.

The day she arrived in Seattle, I picked her up at the air-port and we rushed to the Hutch for a family conference with the doctors. That evening Dad was admitted to a laminar air-flow room which was only 4 by 8 feet. Though it was specifically designed to limit the amount of foreign material in the environment, its confining dimensions caused Dad some discomfort. His chemotherapy and radiation treatments started immediately. It was only a few days before his immune system would be dead, and he was ready to receive a new one from me.

For the first couple of days Dad's attitude was very positive, but as the chemotherapy and radiation treatments began to take their toll on his body, he began to show doubts. At one point he actually said, "I don't know if I can do this."

When Dad's immune system was destroyed, it was now time for me to do my part. Danielle accompanied me to the hospital to have a portion of my bone marrow removed. After I was registered, I put on a hospital gown and lay down on a stretcher. All I could do was smile and laugh. When I get really nervous, I cope by smiling and acting giddy. Danielle was with me the entire time until they took me to the operating room.

The next thing I remember was waking up in a hospital room and finding Danielle sitting next to my bed. They had taken approximately one liter of bone marrow from my body. I wanted to see Dad, so they put me in a wheelchair and Danielle pushed me over to his room. I saw my bone marrow in a plastic bag lying on the counter in the nursing station. He hadn't received it yet.

Danielle and I flew home to Blacksburg the next day. In retrospect, I should have waited a couple more days because, after sitting on the plane for five hours, I had an extensive amount of bruising and soreness in my back. But I missed Danielle and wanted to spend as much time at home with her as I could. Two weeks later I flew back to Seattle to see Dad and to donate blood platelets.

When I arrived at the Hutch and saw my father, there was no longer any doubt that he was sick. I was numb all over. In high school I had volunteered at the hospital where Dad worked. Occasionally my assignments took me to the morgue. In Dad's present condition, I thought he looked like one of the cadavers I had seen there. It is terrible to see someone that you care about look so bad. His hair had fallen out and his body was all swollen and discolored. It was so hard to keep my composure. I said, "Hello Dad," and gave him a hug. Tears started rolling down my face as I sat next to him. Every day was like this for the next few weeks. I wondered how he could keep going. His liver and kidneys began to fail. The doctors told us they were not sure he was going to make it. I donated platelets because his platelet count was critically low. They removed a portion of my platelets for Dad by putting needles and lines in each of my arms. My blood flowed out of one arm through a machine that extracted the platelets. Then the blood was returned to my body through the line in my other arm. Dad responded well to my donated platelets, which made me feel even better about having to go through this procedure repeatedly. His condition was slowly improving.

The first day that he started to have an increasing white cell count was a "red letter" event. This meant that my bone marrow was reproducing in his body. His progress was slow but, viewed over weeks, was an amazing demonstration of how the human body can come back from such a horrific condition.

Once Dad could walk, I walked around the halls at the Hutch with him. I would hold his hand to help support him ... and also just because I loved him. When he was able to fly home, I was brimming over with happiness. Dad had beaten all the odds; he had survived the transplant!

Today, almost three years later, he is back at work, proud

of what he is doing. He is just happy to be alive—something we should all be.

KAREN

After thirteen years, I have finally built up enough courage to put my feelings about my father's illness on paper. Or at least to try. I can remember when my father was admitted to the hospital with pneumonia in 1983; however, the doctors found his condition to be much worse than they had suspected. He had leukemia! We were told that my father didn't have long to live.

From that day on, my family's life would never be the same. For the first few years it wasn't so bad. It really didn't seem as if my dad had a life-threatening illness. He would occasionally get sick; however, in the back of my mind, there was always the fear of what could happen. Because of this, I put a wall between him and myself. Whenever I would think of him dying, I wanted to hurt everyone around me. Inwardly, I was in deep pain. As a result, my mother and father and I went through some very difficult and turbulent times. At one point I even moved in with my grandparents and lived with them for a year but, by my junior year in high school, I had moved back home. My Dad was still doing okay then.

It was a couple of years later before his condition started to worsen and there began to be more and more talk about a transplant. When my Dad would bring up the subject of the transplant and ask my opinion, I never knew what to say. All I knew was that I would get this tight feeling in my throat and my stomach would knot up. I kept thinking, *I don't want to lose you, Dad.*

My mother and father eventually made the decision jointly that he should have a transplant. I didn't think it was a good idea, not wanting my Dad to go through with it when there was such a great chance of his dying. By the time his trans-plant was scheduled, not only were we preparing for this, but also for my brother Scott's wedding.

My brothers and I were tested to see if one of us could be a donor for my Dad. It was determined that both Scott and I could be possible donors. In the end, they decided to use Scott because of the same-sex advantage. Plus, I think Mom and Dad knew that Scott was a lot stronger than I was. I remember thinking that if I donated my marrow to Dad, and he didn't make it, I could never live with myself.

The arrangements were being made for Seattle and the wedding was getting closer and closer. The wedding was so important for Dad to attend. The doctors were pushing him to go to Seattle as soon as possible, but my father insisted on attending Scott's wedding first.

I can remember it being such a happy day. Chris and I were both in the wedding party. When we were standing at the altar and Scott and Danielle were exchanging their vows, I looked over at my Dad. He was crying. I instantly started to also cry and thought, *This is the last time my whole family is going to be together*. Glancing over Danielle's shoulder, I looked at Scott, and he winked at me. It was kind of like he was saying that things were going to be okay.

The reception was beautiful. My parents were so proud and happy as they danced together. I don't think I ever felt so much love among all of us. When I slow danced with Dad, I lost it. I was squeezing him so tightly, praying that this wouldn't be the last time we would dance together. I felt as if everyone was watching us and understanding what we were thinking.

I tried to be so strong the morning Mom and Dad were to fly to Seattle. I left for work before they were to leave. That way it was easier for me. Half way to work, I pulled off to the side of road and began to cry. I wondered, *Would my parents come home together?*

I called my parents very often in Seattle, anxious to find out how they were doing. Later, before Dad was to be admitted to the hospital, Chris and I flew out to Seattle. My younger brother gave me so much support. I don't think he ever knew how much he helped me. Chris, being so strong and calm, kind of kept me together.

At our family conference, the physicians told us what we could expect; however, I never could have imagined what my Dad would have to go through. They took us to his room which was only two doors away from the Dudleys, new friends of my parents. Dad ate his last meal and drank his favorite milk shake before entering the sterile room. This room was so small and confining. Our family is one that is very physical; we love to hug each other but, for now, my father would have to be without hugs. It was sad, thinking about him being so confined. When they hung Scott's bone marrow beside Dad's bed, I prayed, "Just let this work."

My time in Seattle went too fast and soon it was time for me to return home and go to work. It was difficult to leave my father. Dressing in scrub clothes and surgical gloves, I went into his sterile room with him, staying only about ten minutes. I just couldn't take it. I felt so sorry for him and what he was going through. He looked helpless whenever he looked at me. On other visits, I would put my hand through the rubber sleeve in the plastic partition to hold his hand or to just touch him, but I couldn't really feel him. I hated that.

When I was home, it was hard to deal with what was happening in all of our lives. On the telephone with Mom, I would be short and angry. Looking back, I am so sorry for doing that to her. She became the object of my frustrations. In reality, I don't think there is a stronger woman in this world or one who could have been better able to handle what was happening. She cared for my father and was also there for everyone else. I love her so much for what she did for our family.

When Dad needed transfusions of blood platelets, I

returned to Seattle. This was the first time I had donated platelets for him. As I lay on a table, an IV was inserted in each of my arms; the IVs were connected to a machine. After a short time, I sat up on the table and my mother asked me what was wrong. I told her, "The room is vibrating."

She laughed and said, "No Honey, it's just you because you're getting weak." Satisfied with her answer, I allowed myself to feel good that my blood was going to help Dad.

After I donated the platelets, I went over to see him. He had not been able to handle the horribly confining sterile room and they were moving him into another location. The new room had a nice view where he could see the seagulls flying over the city. I knew how important this was to him.

Decorating his room with photographs of our family and friends, and taping all the cards he had received onto the walls was enjoyable for me. I also made posters for his walls which expressed the love of our family.

My heart ached for Dad every time I looked at him and I always cried. At least, I could now touch him and hold him, letting him feel and know how much I loved him.

My Dad and I always thought we had the same color and type of skin, and that our fingers and toes also looked alike. When I was holding his hand; however, I realized that this was no longer true. His fingernails and toenails were coming off and his skin was peeling. I thought, *He can't get any worse.* But he did.

My mother and I stayed with him one night when he was really sick. He was so cold; the three of us were sitting on his bed, holding each other, and shaking from his chills. We kept placing warm blankets around him. *How helpless I felt.* My Mom and I, wearing surgical masks, slept together on a little cot in his room. Wondering how anyone could survive what he was going through, I kept waking up to see if he was okay.

When I had to leave for home again, I said good-bye and walked out in the hallway, feeling empty and scared. A nurse came up to me and said, "You know this might be the last time you'll see your father." I was very upset with her. It was difficult enough for me thinking about Dad, but for someone else to say aloud what I was thinking made me angry.

After I returned home, my Dad's condition worsened before it got better. When he started improving, I was so happy for him and our family. He called me one day and said, "Well Karenie, I guess I am going be able to walk you down the aisle of our church someday after all." I knew then that he would make it home.

Finally the day came! *Mom and Dad were coming home!* I was ecstatic. Waiting to see him walk off the plane was pure torture. I was the first one to hug him and, not wanting to let go, I squeezed him so tightly that he said, "You're going to choke me." Our family was finally back together! Some days are still a battle for my dad, but he gets through each one smiling.

You never want to say that good comes from bad, but this event in my life brought me closer to my parents than I had ever been before. Now, besides being my parents, they are my friends. I hope that, in my marriage, I can be as strong as my mother is in hers.

I love my family so very much!

CHRIS

I can remember arriving at the airport in Seattle where my mother and father were waiting for me. It was a strange feeling, seeing them again, especially in a place that was so foreign to me. It was a place they knew quite well. As we rode to the apartment, I was overwhelmed by the beauty of the city. Yet, despite the surroundings, my mind was focused on the reason we all had gathered thousands of miles from home. The thought of a bone marrow transplant was something that barely, if ever, came up in conversation while my father's leukemia was stable. It had happened so fast and I didn't quite know what to think. My philosophy had always been to enjoy the time my family had together. I thought my father would live a few more years until the leukemia finally took its effect. Although he was fortunate to have lived almost ten years after his diagnosis, a bone marrow transplant now meant the difference between life and death.

We entered the apartment overlooking downtown Seattle. Although we were not able to see Mt. Rainier or Olympic National Park from our windows, outside they were clear for everyone to see. That night I showed the family a video tape I had made from our home movies. It showed we children as we grew into a family. Included in it were songs from old records my parents had saved and these gave a special meaning to each experience. It was important to me that Dad remember all the great times that we had enjoyed together. I knew that there would be a point in time when this would help keep him going. Knowing how important it was for him to go into the transplant with a strong desire to survive and to continue his life with our family, I used the video to help prepare him for his battle.

This was the first time I admitted my uncertainty as to the time, if any, that my family still had together. My father had done so much to prepare himself for this difficult journey, but how were we to prepare ourselves? We were spectators anticipating every moment and hanging on to every new piece of information that was to come along.

The day arrived for Dad to check into the hospital. I remember walking with the video camera in my hand, taping his admission to the Hutch We arrived in my father's room, met his attending physician, and watched him devour a dinner that ended with a milk shake. Little did I know that this was the last food he would be able to eat or drink for quite some time. The treatment had begun, and very quickly I saw it take away the father I had known all my life. He was turned into someone else. I knew he was there inside, underneath all the obvious physical changes that were causing him enormous pain, but it was quite a shock to see his body deteriorate in front of my eyes. The radiation and chemotherapy took their toll on him, making him weak and causing swelling. He slept most of the time and, if he woke up, it was only for a minute or so. However, even when he was awake, he was unable to speak to anyone because of the large doses of medication he taking. All I could do was sit around and watch as we all waited for the bone marrow to grow.

Often, I would sit in one of the waiting rooms where people from other families would also rest and talk. We knew that every day we met again was a good day because it gave us hope. I can vividly recall hearing my father coughing from his room as he vomited, which he did so many times. Sometimes it drove me crazy because there was nothing I could do to help him. I can recall one instance in which he was vomiting blood into a bucket because of the lesions in his mouth and the clots all along his tongue. He received oxygen because many of his organs did not appear to be functioning as they should. All of these events happened within the two weeks that I was in Seattle. In this short time, Dad went from a man with a healthy physical appearance to someone who was battling death. I do not know directly of the events which followed my departure but, from what my mother told me, things got much worse before they got better.

Eventually my brother's bone marrow began to generate itself and Dad showed signs of improvement. Although I had not seen my mother and father for two months, I would eventually greet them again in Seattle along with my father's friend, George. There had been so many events which had transpired since I had left them earlier. My father's recovery had taken many ups and downs. Many times since I left, he had almost died.

On my return to Seattle, I can remember walking into Dad's

room and seeing him in his hospital bed. Because of infections in his blood, he had been readmitted. As I looked at him, I could hardly believe what my eyes were telling me. He was bald and so thin that his sweat pants seemed to have nothing in them. I was so grateful that he was still alive but, at the same time, I was shocked to see what he had become. He looked so weak and fragile, not like the strong father I remembered. We said our good-byes and, as I left the room, I had to stop and sit against the wall in the hallway because I almost fainted. Witnessing these momentous physical changes in my father was one of the hardest things about the entire experience.

A few weeks after I departed from Seattle the second time, my father and mother returned home. They were met by my father's family, our family, and friends. I just couldn't believe he had made it through all that I had seen with my own eyes! My father had been so close to death and seeing him again was the greatest blessing I could ever receive! I'll never forget the feeling that I had when we drove down our street and walked into our house. My father had finally come home!

In the months that passed after his arrival at home, he began the slow struggle to regain his health and strength. His body had been so torn down that it would take years for him to recuperate. Our dinners were usually followed by Dad vomiting in the bathroom. It didn't disgust me at all; it just made me wish that I could help him somehow. Yet these instances slowly vanished from our daily lives and, despite minor physical problems that required him to be hospitalized, my father has now regained much of his health. Sure, he has lost a lot of weight, and physically he will never be quite the same, but he is alive and he is cured. He has returned to work and our family is finally back to normal.

I am so thankful for what the doctors were able to do for my father. Without them, I don't think he would be here today. Yet, my father's success is also due to his attitude in his struggle against leukemia. I am convinced from my experiences in Seattle that if you undergo a transplant thinking you will die, then it is almost inevitable that you will. But if you have the courage to want to live, then your chances for survival are greatly increased. I am thankful that somehow my father found that courage.

Lastly, I would like to add that I prayed for my father all the time. More specifically, I can say that on every birthday, since he was diagnosed, I made a special wish that my father would stay alive and be well. I know there will never be another birthday when I won't continue to wish this. I am just so grateful that God honored my wish and continues to do so.

CHAPTER IX

The Final Steps Back

During the flight home I was excited, but also apprehensive about leaving the medical support services of the Hutch. While there, I always felt my care was in very capable hands. As a former hospital administrator, I was very impressed by every aspect of the healthcare delivery system. In Seattle, because of the number of bone marrow transplants performed at the Hutch, it is not uncommon to see people with bald heads walking around the streets wearing surgical masks. On the plane going home that description fit only me.

As I thought about the other transplant patients who didn't fly home, I was overwhelmed by the events of the past four months. Up until that point, I really hadn't thought about the ordeal that I had endured. As I thanked God for helping me go home, I looked to the sky and made a commitment that during the remainder of my life I would do good things.

As Iva and I departed the plane and walked down the corridor to the airline terminal, I could feel the adrenaline pumping. When I saw our family and friends waiting with noisemakers and signs to welcome us, I realized I was finally home. The trip through the airport and the drive to Greensburg seemed like a dream until we turned onto our street. I had a surge of emotion that sent chills up and down my body as we neared our home. It was appropriate that George and Kathy drove us home because, four months earlier, they had driven us to the same airport to began our odyssey.

Hiedi, our toy poodle, came running out of the house to meet us. There had been many days before the transplant, when I was physically drained by the interferon injections, that Heidi was my only companion. Feeling her jumping against my leg, begging me to pick her up, was her way of saying, "I am glad you're home." Karen had made a welcome home banner that she draped across the second floor windows of the house.

As I walked into our home, I was speechless. I sat down in my favorite chair in the family room and just looked around, thinking about my exercise program and the repetitions that had built my strength before the transplant in order to accomplish this goal. *I had made it back home!*

It is very difficult for me to describe my mental state during the first eighteen months following my transplant. There were many times I wasn't sure my mind would ever regain the thought processes that had previously been mine. Throughout that first winter, I would occasionally fall into lapses of attention where my mind seemed to "shut down." I would stare into space for extended periods of time. Chris told one of his friends that the only thing his father did was sit and watch the weather channel on TV for hours on end. I was on medications to prevent blood clots and seizures and, therefore, was not permitted to drive for six months following our return home. But that was okay; physically and mentally I was not prepared to drive. Due to this limitation, I transferred my medical care to the capable hands of Dr. Terry Evans, a hematologist/oncologist in Greensburg who has followed my progress up until the present.

That winter I took immunosuppressant medications again to control the graft versus-host disease in my mouth. I continued these drugs until I returned to the Hutch for my one-year checkup in the autumn of 1993.

My first year post-transplant is something of a blur due to my decreased mental awareness. The recuperation period was longer than anything I could have imagined. Because I was taking prednisone, I still had the moon face of a transplant patient. My hair started coming back in November and by Christmas I looked as though I had a crew cut. At church on Christmas Eve, I needed to sit down as our fellow parishioners greeted us following the service. I wondered whether I would ever feel normal again.

When I began driving once more in the spring of 1993, I had barely enough strength in my legs to operate the brake pedal. Aware of my physical limitations, I was very cautious. Because I drove so slowly, I always had a string of cars following me.

In that same spring, I began exercising again at the Aerobic Center of Greensburg. This was the facility that had prepared me so well for the transplant. It was good to see Assad, a trainer at the facility, who had designed my successful program of free weights and strengthening machines during my preparation for the transplant. But the spirit and inspiration behind the creation of the Aerobic Center is Eddie Hutchinson, ex-marine and Greensburg city fire chief, a one-of-a-kind individual. He would pump me up with enthusiasm by just being around him. "Hutch" showed up at my door with an exercise bicycle given to me by an anonymous donor the day after I returned from Seattle. He told me later that he said to a friend as they were leaving the house that day, "I've seen dead people who look better than Jack does." He always had a unique way with words. I enjoyed the look of amazement on his face as he watched me exercising in the summer of 1993.

As I began to strengthen my body, I started a program to strengthen my mind. At first I would read a sentence and then try to recite it in my head. As I became more and more proficient, I would attempt entire paragraphs. This process began in the summer of 1993 and continued into the autumn. As I continued my mental training, I noticed I was becoming more alert and aware of my surroundings. Staring less and less, with my lapses of attention decreasing, I moved on to taking my son's sample college entrance exams.

I always tried to hide my mental deficit from those around me. College financial aid documents for Chris were submitted three times before they were deemed acceptable. I couldn't tell him that I was unable to concentrate long enough to read and complete the questions. I couldn't accept the notion that in surviving the transplant I had become a mental cripple. My short-term memory was my biggest problem so I constantly repeated names, dates, and so on, in my mind, so I would not forget the information.

Although my progress was slow those first twelve months, I improved both physically and mentally and was excited about my return trip to Seattle in October 1993 for my one-year post-transplant checkup.

The name Seattle will always conjure up pleasant memories in my mind. I couldn't wait to visit the Hutch and see the nurses and the staff. As I walked into the facility, my heart was pounding. This was the place that had helped me begin my second life. As I hugged each nurse, I realized how important this return visit was to my recovery. It was a crucial step in the healing process. There is a level of satisfaction in visiting the same places where you once were so weak that you could barely walk and, upon returning, felt like running along those same hallways and sidewalks.

During the visit, the nurses escorted me to several patient rooms. I would stand in the doorway while the nurse gave the patient a brief history of my transplant experience and then would say, "And see how good he looks now."

All of my follow-up tests were performed at an outpatient facility, but Iva and I visited the Hutch many times during our stay. I wanted to make sure I saw and thanked all the people who helped me through the transplant. One of the persons who appreciated seeing me as much as I appreciated seeing him was the nurse who performed my dialysis when my kidneys failed. He commented that most of the patients he treated were seriously ill and that very few ever returned for follow-up visits.

On one of my visits to the Hutch, a lady approached me. She seemed hesitant. "I—I hope that I'm not being too forward but my mother saw you yesterday and told me that you are a former bone marrow transplant patient. Is that true?"

"Yes, I'm back for my one-year checkup. How may I help you?"

"She said you were laughing and that you look great — and she's right. Is there a possibility that you could talk to my husband? He just received a transplant and needs some encouragement. We all do!"

"Of course," I said. "I know about the importance of encouragement."

When I saw the sores on his lips, it reminded me of what I had gone through. I kept assuring him that things would get better. They had gotten better for me.

It was during one of these visits to the Hutch that the head nurse confided in me that, at one point during my hospitalization, I was the sickest patient they had at that time on the unit. When I was discharged, she and the other nurses said I was a survivor. Enthusiastically, I described to her what I had done to keep myself alive.

Her response surprised me. "Take the time to document your experiences regarding the leukemia and transplant. Your words could provide inspiration for other people facing life-threatening illnesses."

"I'll—I'll think about it," I said. And I did. Her comments inspired the writing of this book.

During our last visit to the Hutch, I asked Iva to give me a moment to myself. I couldn't leave without walking around the unit one more time. But I wanted to walk alone, celebrating the fact that I didn't need the physical support of Iva or the children. I had tears of joy in my eyes and the same feeling of exhilaration that I had the day I completed that same walk a year earlier.

Before, during, and after my transplant, Iva was the stable rock that kept the family going. I never saw her show the emotional strain she was under while I was in Seattle for my transplant. On our follow-up visit, however, as we were leaving the Hutch, she went over and sat down on a bench and began to cry. When I asked what was wrong, she said, "I've kept this in for a year." Visiting the Hutch had brought her suppressed emotions to the surface.

In the first year following my return home from the transplant, I was hospitalized twice: initially for pneumonia that first winter, and then for a kidney stone in the spring of 1993. Having been told that I had developed cataracts from the radiation treatments I had received prior to the transplant, I, subsequently had lens implants in both eyes in 1994. Presently, I continue to take medication to prevent kidney stones. My strength continues to increase.

A couple of weeks before we initially left for Seattle, my friend George and I were sitting on a bench in my back yard, discussing the anxieties and emotions of my family as we approached this unknown event in our lives. George surprised me with the comment, "I wonder what type of person you'll be when you return home?"

I immediately responded, "I hope I'm the same person that I am now." I had never thought about the possibility of changes in my personality as a result of what I was about to experience. But George's insight was to prove correct. I think Iva said it best when she told me that I left a little bit of myself in Seattle. One part of me that I left there was my ability to meditate. I have tried many times but cannot duplicate the

134

meditation process that I had used so successfully through the years prior to my transplant. For me, it is as if I had a few layers of my personality stripped away and, each day post-transplant, I am adding again to the depth of my personality.

During my life I have been blessed with the friendship of some very special people. One of these individuals is P.J. Jannetta M.D., Chairman of the Department of Neurosurgery at the University of Pittsburgh. During my follow-up visit to the Hutch, it was discovered that I had a small brain infarction (stroke). When I returned home, I scheduled an appointment with P.J. to review the brain scans performed in Seattle. In the end, the brain infarction proved to be a minor nuisance because it only affects my ability to perform fine motor functions. (I don't attempt to untangle Iva's chain necklaces anymore.)

During my appointment with P.J., he asked me what my plans were, saying that he wanted me to do some consulting work for the Department of Neurosurgery.

I said, "I'm not sure what I'm capable of doing."

He looked at me intensely. "During your hospitalization, following the transplant, I received a call from a neurosurgical resident at the University of Washington who told me that you probably wouldn't survive more than a few days."

"Surviving was part of my plan," I said. "I couldn't give up —my family was always before me."

"You're a fighter and you won. You beat the odds. You're the kind of person I want on my team—someone who can accomplish whatever they set out to do."

P.J. is an individual who possesses a genuine goodness in his dealings with his fellow man and in his approach to life. I will always be grateful to him for giving me the opportunity to complete the rebuilding of my thought processes. In July 1994, I accepted the position of Executive Administrator for the Department of Neurosurgery.

My blessings continued. Eleven years after I had become

ill, I completed the cycle, returning to my original place of employment. A portion of my journey back was complete.

My friend Scott Dudley continues to do well. We have made an effort to visit each other every few months. Iva and I either drive to Indiana or Scott and Jeanne drive to Pennsylvania. Most frequently, we meet halfway in Columbus, Ohio, for a two-day visit. One of my friends joked that it's like two military veterans getting together to exchange war stories. We continue to telephone each other every few weeks to update the events in our lives. Conversations about our transplants have decreased over time since we left Seattle. Today, there is a relationship between the four of us that is difficult to describe. It is more than a bond between friends; it is like the bond that exists between members of a family.

I often think about the blessings in my life. By living nine years with chronic myelocytic leukemia, I lived into the last five percent of the survival curve with my type of illness. My bone marrow transplant was successful even though the odds of my survival were one in five. I have been so blessed and often ask why I survived when fellow patients who were younger and stronger with fewer complications didn't make it.

A few months ago, I was speaking to a group of seminarians who were training to become hospital chaplains. Following my presentation, I commented that God must have something He wants me to do in this life and I wished He would tell me what it was. The reply of one young seminarian, startled me. "Maybe you are already doing it," he said with all sincerity.

When I remember my summer in Seattle, I remember it with a smile on my face. In my mind, I cannot visualize a more pleasurable place to experience what I had to endure. Having once heard that happiness is the ability to selectively forget, I can say, " I don't remember the pain. However, I do remember the beautiful Northwest, the great staff at the Hutch, our fun times with the Dudley's, and most of all, the support of our friends and family."

My journey back from leukemia and the transplant ended January 4, 1995, in Richmond, Virginia when a daughter was born to Danielle and Scott. This fulfilled the final commitment that I had made at their wedding. Holding my granddaughter in my arms, I said, "Welcome to the world Summer Anne; I am your grandfather and I love you."